The Anywhere, Anytime Chill Guide

The Anywhere, Anytime Chill Guide

77 Simple Strategies for Serenity

Kate Hanley,
Ms. Mindbody

Guilford, Connecticut
An imprint of The Globe Pequot Press

To buy books in quantity for corporate use
or incentives, call **(800) 962–0973**
or e-mail **premiums@GlobePequot.com.**

 is an attitude . . . spirited, independent, outspoken, serious, playful and irreverent, sometimes controversial, always passionate.

Illustrations by Béatrice Favereau | www.beatricefavereau.com
Text design by Sheryl P. Kober

Library of Congress Cataloging-in-Publication Data
Hanley, Kate.
 The anywhere, anytime chill guide : 77 simple strategies for serenity / Kate Hanley.
  p. cm.
 ISBN 978-1-59921-393-4
1. Stress management. I. Title.
 RA785.H367 2009
 616.9'8—dc22

2008012877

Printed in the United States of America
10 9 8 7 6 5 4 3 2 1

For Scott, my ultimate sanity saver

Contents

Contents

Contents

Contents

Acknowledgments

Oddly enough, my initial thanks go to Oliver Stone and Alan Parker, who respectively wrote and directed *Midnight Express*—my first exposure to yoga. Seeing the main character perform a Sun Salutation convinced me that if yoga could help inmates handle life in a Turkish prison, it could also help me feel . . . what, exactly, I didn't know. I only knew it would be better. That one scene, watched thirteen years ago, started me on the path that has ultimately led to writing this book.

Heaps of gratitude to Mary Norris, Lara Asher, and Imee Curiel at Skirt! for believing in this project and in me, and for their graceful guidance throughout the publishing process; my agent, Stephanie Kip Rostan, who stuck by me through several book ideas and who never wavered in her support; and Marian Lizzi, whose well-timed and generous encouragement helped me persevere when I was growing weary of searching for a publishing home. Sincere thanks also to MP Dunleavey and Amy Paturel for their careful reading of an early draft and their spot-on suggestions.

I hate to even contemplate what my writing life would be like without my support group of fellow writers. They generously share their knowledge, camaraderie, and overall brilliance, and make this otherwise solitary profession feel like a great group adventure.

My immeasurable thanks to all my teachers, past and present, particularly Kristen Davis, Witold Fitz-Simon, and Deborah Wolk at the Yogasana Center in Brooklyn. They have helped me see how subtle adjustments can yield profound results. My appreciation extends especially to Witold for his support, suggestions, and enthusiasm for this book. And perhaps most importantly, I give my humblest thanks to my teachers' teach-ers. None of what's contained in these pages would still be in use today if a few people didn't learn everything they could about these disciplines and then share their knowledge with others. If you find something here that works particularly well for you (and I sincerely hope you do), pass it on.

Introduction

The phone is ringing, you've just received an annoying e-mail from a coworker, there's a big meeting in ten minutes, and your stomach is in knots. What do you do? Take two hours to go to a yoga class? Book a massage? Take a swig from the emergency flask you keep in the top right-hand drawer?

Here in the real world, you've got two choices: A) Ignore the crick in your neck, wash your rising panic down with coffee and a leftover pastry you find in the office kitchen, and forge ahead, hoping the sugar crash doesn't come too quickly. Or B), take half a minute to do a simple stretch that will release your tight muscles, a breathing exercise that allows the body to let go of stress, or a quick meditation technique that will quiet your swirling thoughts, so you can go into that meeting with a clear head and an energized body.

Simply put, you can perpetuate your misery, or you can take a step toward feeling better. Which one will it be?

Most of us would like to choose feeling better. After all, that's the impulse that has us reaching for junk food, java, and a daily glass (or three) of red wine. But we know too much about health to continue justifying these choices that may provide a quick fix, but ultimately perpetuate feelings of exhaustion, irritability, and overall upset. The problem is, most people don't realize how easy it is to take better care of themselves, even in the midst of a messy, messed-up, million-mile-an-hour day.

Luckily, humans have been perfecting elemental self-care techniques for millennia. Yogis, practitioners of traditional Chinese medicine, and herbalists all have a vast arsenal of simple things that are specifically designed to remedy ailments of the body, mind, and spirit. This book is an easy-to-follow guide to using these ancient practices in the midst of even the crappiest day—no turbans, incense, or two-week spa visits required. Its goal is to empower you to take steps each and every day toward becoming calmer, more resilient, and happier, even when life is at its most chaotic.

I know what you're probably thinking: How can she possibly expect me to find the time to do these things? And do they even work anyway? I've addressed these concerns below:

Concern No. 1:
"I'm already way too busy, how can I add even one more thing to my daily to-do list?"

Answer: I have specifically chosen remedies that will work even if you only do them for a breath or two. (Of course, longer is more restful, but a little bit of feeling good is always better than none.)

If I suggest you try a remedy for five minutes, and the very thought of taking that much time only adds to your stress levels, try it for one minute instead. If even a minute seems too long, aim for thirty seconds. The most important thing is that you try it. First, merely setting an intention to take better care of yourself starts you on the path to building your self-care muscles. Then, once you create the conditions for your mind and body to relax, you'll likely enjoy it and stay a little longer. And once you see how much better you feel when you try a natural remedy when you would otherwise reach for a cigarette, piece of candy, or can of soda, maybe you'll be inspired to practice them more regularly.

Concern No. 2:
"How can something as simple as the remedies you suggest actually work?"

Answer: If taking fifteen seconds to pause and take a deep breath helps you handle stress more gracefully—even if it's only an *iota* of extra grace—it's worth it. According to the scientific principle of inertia, an object in motion has a tendency to stay in motion and an object at rest has the tendency to stay at rest. By the same principle, moving even a hair toward feeling better breeds more upward progression. I'll bet you've witnessed the opposite—a self-created downward spiral—in your own life: One morning, you stubbed your toe on the way to bathroom. You howled and got cranky. Then in the kitchen, you cut your finger while slicing a banana for your cereal. By the time you left the house, you were downright surly. And wouldn't you know it—that was the day you found a parking ticket on your car?

I'm not suggesting you instantly transform into Pollyanna Happypants and smile serenely in the face of every obstacle. Sadly, no remedy or combination of remedies in this book will solve all your problems. (I am so sorry to be the bearer of bad news. If you'd like to return the book and get your money back, I'll understand.) You will still get riled when your computer crashes moments before you're due to deliver an important presentation. But you can choose how you react to inevitable frustrations and whether you allow them to ruin the rest of your day. If you take a moment to give your mind and body what it needs to stay thoughtful instead of reactionary, such as an easy stretch that banishes tension, you'll be 1,000 times more likely to choose a course of action that mitigates the situation rather than escalates it. With a little practice, you'll be able to smooth out the curves in your daily stress roller coaster. And when this happens, the benefits ripple throughout the rest of your life—you sleep more soundly, have more energy, become less prone to mood swings, and generally enjoy life a little more.

Concern No. 3:
"What kind of impact can these physical exercises have on my mental state?"

Answer: Although stress may seem like a phenomenon that's strictly mental, it is actually the result of a number of processes that take place throughout the body. When we experience something that causes us mental or emotional stress, our bodies secrete hormones, such as adrenaline, that actually cause physiological changes that add up to "feeling bad"—airways constrict, muscles tighten, digestion slows, and the heart races. Many of the remedies in this book work to alleviate these physical symptoms, which in turn induces the body's relaxation response, reduces the swells of an emotional storm, and leads to "feeling better."

About Me

Although I am a certified yoga teacher, I am not a yoga goddess or a guru. I cannot levitate, control my heart rate with my mind, or do a handstand in the middle of the room. (Yet.)

I am a dedicated student of yoga and seeker of simple things we can all do to feel better in our minds, bodies, and souls. I have practiced the self-care techniques described in this book in the midst of cross-country moves, tragic breakups, insane workloads, and—perhaps my biggest challenge yet—the transition to motherhood. I've learned that while it's not always easy to put your well-being first, even small, simple steps can have profound results. And I'm passionate about sharing what I'm constantly discovering with people who are curious about what they can do to feel less frazzled and more fulfilled.

How to Use This Book

Since it's designed to help you in the midst of even your busiest day, this book is ridiculously easy to use. Arranged by subject, and inspired by the tried-and-true cookbook format, it gives concise instructions for simple practices, or "remedies," that meet very particular needs. Each remedy has an ingredient list, an amount of time needed, and step-by-step instructions. Each remedy is also cross-referenced to other remedies that can help you deal with that particular situation, where appropriate. For example, the remedy for menstrual cramps—a simple seated forward bend where your forehead rests on a chair—can also alleviate headaches, so I've listed "Supported Seated Forward Bend" under the "Other Remedies to Try" section of the entry on headaches. If you try any remedy and are still looking for relief, refer to those other remedies for further guidance.

When you find yourself in a stinky situation, look it up in the index for quick access. Or read a particular section when you're experiencing an uptick in challenges in that part of your life. Or just read a remedy or two each day so you can be prepared when the crap hits the fan.

And for continuing inspiration, visit MsMindbody.com, where I post regular columns that describe simple techniques you can use to pursue the fine art of feeling better and better.

Take care and keep breathing,

Kate

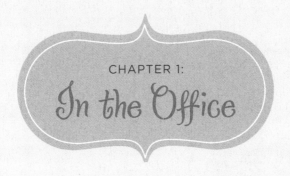

CHAPTER 1:

In the Office

The office is the perfect place to practice simple stress-reducing techniques because, let's face it, it's one of the most stressful places on Earth: This is where your buttons get pushed as hard as they can be pushed *and* where you're always expected to act with composure and professionalism. When you have an important presentation coming up, or your boss shoots down one of your ideas in a big meeting, or your computer crashes, you can't huff and puff, cry, or chug a glass of wine—these tactics simply aren't the viable options here that they are in the privacy of your own home. Perhaps, with a little practice, the techniques in this chapter will actually help you begin to loosen up a little more at work. You spend the majority of your waking hours on the clock—you may as well enjoy them.

This is where your buttons get pushed as hard as they can be pushed.

Job Interview

It's a big day for you. You have an opportunity to present your experience and your unique "you-ness." And if things go well, you could receive a job offer that will change your daily reality in a major way. It's time to bring your A game.

> You want to keep your wits about you so that you can wow 'em.

You want to keep your wits about you so that you can wow 'em with your confidence and smarts. But you can't be all drive and focus; you also need to remain open and receptive in order to gather as much information about your potential new employer as you convey about yourself. After all, since you'd spend most of your waking hours toiling away for them, you want to make sure it's a good fit.

This exercise will calm you and clear your head so that you speak eloquently, think on your feet, and take in subtle clues about what it would actually feel like to work for this place. Do it before you leave the house, or in your car before you head in for the meeting. ✿

Remedy:
Alternate Nostril Breathing

Ingredients:
Quiet
Privacy

Time Needed:
One to five minutes

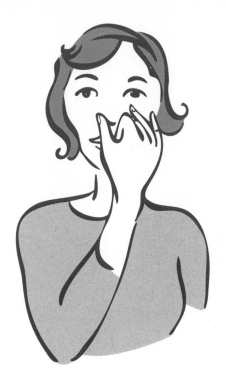

Instructions:

◎ Sit any which way you can comfortably support a tall spine, such as cross-legged on the floor with your back resting against a wall or in a straight-backed chair with both feet firmly on the floor.

◎ Fold the index and middle fingers of your right hand into your palm.

◎ Bring your right palm up in front of your face and rest the ring finger on the left side of your nose and the thumb on the right side of your nose, just underneath the bony bridge.

🌀 Gently press your thumb to block your right nostril and inhale a breath through your left nostril.

🌀 Release your thumb, press your ring finger to close off your left nostril, and exhale through the right nostril.

🌀 Keep your fingers the same and inhale through the right nostril.

🌀 Switch your fingers to exhale through the left nostril.

🌀 Continue breathing this way, exhaling and inhaling through one nostril at a time, for up to five minutes.

🌀 End with an exhale through the left nostril.

🌀 Take a few normal breaths before you return to your day.

Modifications:

🌀 Use a light touch. You need to press just firmly enough to temporarily block the flow of air. You don't want to traumatize your delicate nasal passages.

🌀 It's all about slow and steady in this exercise—refrain from sucking in the air as if it were your last breath.

🌀 Each inhale and exhale should be roughly the same length. If it helps, silently count to four during each breath. If that adds one too many layers of complexity, skip it and simply do your best.

🌀 This exercise works well anytime you need to be simultaneously focused and relaxed, such as when asking for a raise, having a difficult conversation, working on a project, or spending time with someone who pushes your buttons. It's a great tool to have in your arsenal.

Benefits:

◎ Alternate nostril breathing activates both sides of the brain evenly, enabling you to bring your full range of mental capabilities with you into the interview: creative and logical, intuitive and analytical, passionate and rational.

◎ Such careful attention to the breath calms the mind and promotes relaxation, so that you can be yourself during the interview instead of tongue-tied and nervous.

◎ Blocking one nostril at a time forces the lungs to work harder than normal. As a result, this breath brings more oxygen into the body, gently energizing it. Meaning you can go in there and dazzle them with your vibrance.

> **Other Remedies to Try:**
> Arms Up, Chest Up • Get Grounded

Oversleeping

hoops. You've slept right through the alarm and now you need to get up and out the door in record time. First things first: Everyone oversleeps sometimes. Don't waste any of your precious energy and limited time on beating yourself up. Drama is a luxury only the idle can afford—have you ever seen any of the characters in soap operas working hard?

Your best strategy is to make yourself presentable as quickly as you can and reserve as much time as possible for making sure you leave the house with everything you need for the day—which includes breakfast. Yes, time is precious. Of course you don't want to go to work with a rat's nest for hair. But it's better to sport a ponytail and have a full belly (not to mention your calendar, cell phone, and wallet) than it is to have a perfect coif, a growling stomach, and no money for lunch.

If you don't have the ingredients on hand for this recipe, you can find them at practically any food store—even 7-Eleven carries fruit and nuts. By the time eleven o'clock rolls around, you will be so thankful you took those few minutes to give your body the fuel it needs.

Remedy:
A Filling and Energizing Breakfast (you can eat on the go)

Ingredients:
Apple or pear
Handful of raw nuts, such as almonds or cashews

Time Needed:
Ninety seconds to wash and dry the fruit
and put the nuts in a baggie
Five minutes to eat

Instructions:

◎ Grab an apple or pear and give it a quick scrub under running water. Dry it with a kitchen towel.

◎ Take a handful of nuts and throw them in a baggie.

◎ Run out the door.

◎ You can eat your no-time-for-breakfast breakfast in the car, on the bus or train, or even at your desk (if your coworkers don't mind the sound of crunching).

Modifications:

◎ If you actually have time to sit down for two minutes before you head out the door, core and slice the apple or pear and eat it with a healthy shmear of peanut, cashew, or almond butter. It's delicious and has the same benefits.

Benefits:

◎ The fiber in the apple or pear keeps you full for much longer than its less-than-100 calories might suggest.

◎ The protein in the nuts boosts your stores of energy.

◎ The nuts also contain fiber and healthy fats. They will also help you stay full until you have time for a proper meal.

◎ You'll have the benefit of knowing that you've taken steps to give your body what it needs to function well.

Other Remedies to Try:
Hot/Cold Water Therapy • Ring the Gong

Crowded Elevator

You may have a natural aversion to small spaces, or you may never give your average, uncrowded elevator ride a second thought. But get ten or more bodies in one slow-moving elevator and you've got a recipe for some serious mental discomfort.

Being on a crowded elevator is yet another way that the universe shows you that you are not in full control: You can't reach the button, there's no corner to retreat into, you have no idea how many times you'll have to stop before you get to your destination. But it's also a great reminder that everyone is in this thing called "life" together. Someone will have to push the button for you, someone else will likely step on your toe by accident, the guy's stomach in the back will be rumbling. Oh, the humanity!

> It's a great reminder that everyone is in this thing called "life" together.

You need to keep your cool and give yourself something to think about other than how many floors you have to suffer through before you can step off. You also need to stay loose to accommodate the changing gravity, and open, so that you can relate to your fellow passengers and survive this tight spot as members of the same team. This exercise helps you take your thoughts away from how little control you have as it creates more space and stability in your body.

Remedy:
Neck Lift

Ingredients:
N/A

Time Needed:
As long as necessary

Instructions:

- Start by feeling both of your feet planted firmly on the floor, your heels and toes reaching down with equal weight.

- In your mind, find the uppermost part of the back of your neck—the soft spot just underneath the pointy part of your skull. This is the very top of your spine, and lies directly behind your ears.

- Subtly lift this part of your spine straight up toward the ceiling. It doesn't have to be a large movement; it's more a point of focus that will have a moderate effect on the body.

- Let the back of your neck be so light that the spine lengthens naturally, as if your head were a balloon and your spine were the string attached to it.

- Notice how much more room you now have in your chest and abdomen.

- Also check to see if your posture has affected the people around you. Often, taller posture is contagious, like a yawn.

- Each time you find that you've slumped back down, simply start again.

Modifications:
N/A

Benefits:

🌀 Helps you expand your presence, which gives you the illusion of having more space

🌀 Creates more room in your torso, enabling you to breathe more deeply

🌀 Strengthens your core muscles

🌀 Encourages better posture

🌀 Gives your mind something to focus on, which is relaxing

🌀 Can also be practiced nearly anywhere—walking down the street, driving, sitting at your desk, standing in the kitchen making scrambled eggs. . . .

Other Remedies to Try:
The Human Tape Recorder • Stress Scan

Procrastinating

You have a huge list of things to accomplish, but your stores of motivation are woefully small. It's enough to make you want to shake your fist at the sky. Or become engrossed in the state of your cuticles. Or decide that now is the perfect time to catch up on all the gossip Web sites. Anything to distract you from doing whatever it is that needs your attention.

Procrastination is like mold—ignore it and it will grow. The one thing that has the power to deflate it is action. Even taking one small step to get started can help snap you out of procrastination's spell. This exercise purges all the lame excuses your cunning mind can devise and leaves you energized and ready to focus. Prepare to kick some major butt! 🌺

Remedy:
Powerful Breath

Ingredients:
Chair (preferably straight-backed)

Time Needed:
One minute

Instructions:

◉ Sit on the edge of your chair with your feet resting flat on the floor.

◉ Lift the back of your neck up toward the ceiling to lengthen your spine.

◉ Breathing through your nose with your mouth closed, take one deep inhale and one full exhale.

◎ Continuing to breathe through your nose, inhale a normal breath.

◎ Exhale quickly and forcefully through your nose, as if you were trying to blow out a birthday candle. As you do so, draw your belly button in toward your spine.

◎ Release your stomach muscles and allow your next inhale to flow effortlessly through your nasal passages. This completes one breath.

◎ Take several breaths this way—aim for between five and twenty.

Modifications:

◎ What's happening with your belly is equally as important as what's happening with your nose. Proceed as slowly as you like until you get the hang of the active exhale (when the belly draws in) and the passive inhale (when the belly releases).

Benefits:

◎ Powerful breathing clears impurities out of the sinus and nasal cavities and promotes clearer thinking and heightened awareness. This exercise in Sanskrit is known as *kapalabhati*, which translates to "skull-shining breath." The idea is that you're breathing so vigorously you can clear any cobwebs right out of your head.

◎ Stimulates the digestive system. All that in and out with your belly button wakes up your entire abdomen—the source of your personal power—and gets things moving down there.

◎ You will release any tension you may be holding in your diaphragm and encourage your breath to deepen. So while you're clearing out and waking up, you're also promoting relaxation, meaning you'll be able to calmly allow the inspiration to flow instead of trying to force it.

◎ You'll feel invigorated, both mentally and physically.

> **Other Remedies to Try:**
> Head Down Time Out
> One-Minute Visualization
> Plank Pose

Work Avalanche

There will inevitably be times when your workload—and your stress level—skyrockets. You can deal with the influx by increasing your daily dose of caffeine and/or cigarettes, succumbing to the temptation of comforting yourself with sweet or salty snacks, or depriving yourself of sleep in the name of making it through the tough times at any cost.

The sticky wicket is that all those things that you do because they seem as if they're going to make you feel better or give you energy will actually only make you feel worse. Chugging coffee will leave you jittery and impede your ability to sleep well later that night. Smoking cigarettes only gives your already overtaxed body more toxins to process and store.

Eating lots of oh-so-delicious but nutritionally bereft snacks doesn't give your body—or your brain—the fuel it needs to support you in your time of need. And neglecting sleep makes it harder for your body to recover from the day, can disrupt your hormonal balance, and has a direct impact on your cognitive function. On top of that, you are too valuable a resource to completely deplete yourself in the name of work. You won't do anyone any good—yourself, your family, your employer, or your clients—if you are an exhausted shell of a woman.

> *You are too valuable a resource to completely deplete yourself in the name of work.*

So what's an insanely busy gal to do? It's simple: Give your body what it needs. Eat a healthy breakfast of whole grains, protein, and fresh fruit so that even if the rest of your food day is a disaster, you'll at least have some nutrition in you. Get some fresh air, even if it's only a ten-minute walk around the block after eating lunch at your desk in front of the computer. Give yourself thirty minutes of quiet time before you go to bed—no TV, no phone calls, no loud music—so that you have a little time to wind down and set the stage for sleep. (You could spend this time massaging your feet, taking a bath, reading a book, or stepping outside to look at the stars—all easy ways to relax.)

If you do need a stronger boost of energy, the following homeopathic remedy is specifically designed to help you through hectic, emotionally trying times. Its primary ingredients are the essences of flowers that have been extracted by steeping or boiling them in spring water. Each flower was chosen for its purported effect on emotions: impatiens (encourages patience and empathy), star-of-Bethlehem (eases trauma), cherry plum (boosts intuition and confidence), rock rose (reduces panic), and clematis (promotes clear thinking). By tucking a tiny bottle of this all-natural remedy in your purse—or stashing it in your desk drawer—and taking it regularly until the storm has passed, you'll be giving yourself something completely natural, noncaloric, and nonaddictive to reach for when you need a little metaphorical shot in the arm. 🌸

Remedy:
Rescue Remedy

Ingredients:
A bottle of Rescue Remedy
(purchased at any health food store)

Time Needed:
Once you have a bottle on hand, mere seconds

Instructions:
◎ Place three to four drops of Rescue Remedy under your tongue and let them absorb naturally.

◎ That's it!

◎ You can repeat up to four times a day until you're feeling more like your normal, not-ruled-by-stress self.

Modifications:
◎ You can also place two drops in a glass of water and sip it as you need it.

◎ Bach Flower Essences, the manufacturer of Rescue Remedy, makes several different forms of the potion—you can also buy it as a spray, or as a small, dissolvable tablet known as a pastille. If you don't like the drops under your tongue, try another form until you find one that works well for you.

Benefits:

◉ Alleviates impatience

◉ Increases your ability to recover from setbacks

◉ Helps you disengage from drama and trust your inner wisdom

◉ Reduces anxiety

◉ Promotes clarity

◉ Helps you achieve more restful sleep so that you can wake up tomorrow and do it all over again

Other Remedies to Try:
Chamomile Tea
Legs Up the Wall
Supported Child's Pose

Looming Deadlines

You have a major project with a firm deadline. You know it's time to focus, but for some reason you just . . . can't . . . get . . . started. There are so many things on your to-do list that you can't figure out where to begin. And there are sooooo many fun sites to surf on the Internet. Then you have e-mails to read, voice mails to return, and decisions to make about your next meal. When you're finally ready to dive in, chatty Patty stops by your cube, or you get called into a meeting, or the phone rings.

Although life will always have legitimate curveballs to throw our way, we're often our own worst enemies. We can find any number of cockamamie excuses not to do something. What we need is some inspiration for getting things done.

This exercise helps you put the substantial power of your mind to work for you instead of against you. It's a super-simple visualization that encourages you to embrace the notion that things can be easy. Rather than forcing yourself into getting started through sheer will alone, blaze a mental trail that you can easily follow. ❀

Remedy:
One-Minute Visualization

Ingredients:
Enough privacy for you to feel comfortable
closing your eyes

Time Needed:
Sixty seconds
(although you can continue for as long as it's helpful)

Instructions:

◎ Sit comfortably in a chair. You can also lie on the couch if you have one of those fancy corner offices (or a home office).

◎ Close your eyes and, for a few moments, listen to the soothing sound of your own breath.

◎ Think of releasing tension each time you exhale.

◎ After several breaths, begin to visualize yourself doing everything it will take for you to meet your deadline. Imagine yourself working effortlessly, finding just the right piece of information or tool you need right when you need it, even enjoying the process as your best work naturally bubbles to the surface.

◎ Be as specific as you can. Feel your fingers flying across the keyboard, for example, and notice how relaxed your body feels when you are working "in the zone."

◎ Finally, see yourself finishing with plenty of time to spare. Imagine how good it feels to complete a job well done. Savor this delicious feeling.

◎ Gently open your eyes and sit quietly for a few beats before you get busy.

Modifications:

◎ Write down your visualization instead of letting all the action occur in your head. Start by writing, "I can see myself . . ." and then continue by recording all the tasks you'll be able to complete and how you'll feel while you're doing them. (This approach has the added benefit of helping you look busy to your coworkers and boss.)

◎ You can use this technique in a variety of situations to help ensure that things go smoothly—having a difficult conversation, trying something new, or any activity that causes your anxiety levels to start rising.

Benefits:

◎ Helps you focus on exactly what you need to do

◎ Relaxes your body so that you can do it with a minimum of stress

◎ Improves your powers of concentration

◎ Promotes feelings of well-being when your tendency may be to mentally berate yourself

Other Remedies to Try:
Head Down Time Out • Powerful Breath

Stuck on Hold

There you are, cruising through your workday, when you get placed on hold during a routine call. (Cue the corny music.) Suddenly everything screeches to a halt. You have to sit still, attached to your phone. And worse yet, you have no idea how long you'll be there. The pain! And no, you can't solve the problem by placing the call on speakerphone and subjecting everyone in the office to the hold music. That's just rude.

> *You can use this forced time out as a rare occasion to consciously relax.*

There is something you can do, however. You can use this forced time out as a rare occasion to consciously relax. Left to its own devices, your mind might naturally take this opportunity to think of all the many things stressing you out. But you can gently coax its attention toward a much more beneficial and productive task—sniffing around for hidden spots of stress and chasing them out of town, kind of like a sheriff in an old Western movie.

Remedy:
Stress Scan

Ingredients:
Attention

Time Needed:
As long as you're stuck on hold . . .

Instructions:

◉ Resist the urge to slump over your desk in despair and instead sit up nice and tall. Scoot back so that you can rest your spine on the back of your chair.

◉ Hold the phone in your hand instead of craning your neck and hunching your shoulder to keep the handset in place (or better yet, switch to a headset).

◉ Place both feet flat on the floor.

◉ Start by focusing your attention on your head and jaw. Scan the area to search for any pockets of tension hiding up there, which may show up as a clenching in your jaw, or a furrow in your brow, or even a subtle frown on your lips. You're looking for any muscles that are tight, hard, or straining.

◉ With each exhale, imagine any stress you find dissipating.

◉ Continue by methodically working your way down your entire body—neck, shoulders, chest, arms, stomach, hips, buttocks, thighs, calves, and feet.

◉ Spend three to five breaths focusing on each area, scanning, breathing, and releasing.

◉ When you finish, start again. Each time you move through the body, you'll be able to uncover deeper layers of stress and create more opportunities to relax.

Modifications:

◉ You can keep this up as long as they can keep you on hold. You'll simply get more and more relaxed.

◎ You can also use this technique on a head-clearing walk around the block, as you're waiting at the doctor's office, or any time you have a few mental moments to yourself that might otherwise be an invitation to think about your to-do list.

Benefits:

◎ Keeps your brain occupied so that your body can relax

◎ Helps you use this annoying and unavoidable part of modern life to your benefit

◎ Improves focus, so that when you finally do get to speak to someone, you'll be better able to ask for what you need

◎ Creates a mini oasis of relaxation in even the busiest day

Other Remedies to Try:
4-7-8 Breath • Seated Spinal Twist

Public Speaking

For some people, public speaking is no big deal. If you are one of these people, this recipe is not for you! Go take a walk outside and revel in your non-neurosis.

This is for those of you whose hearts start palpitating and palms start sweating at the mere thought of getting up in front of a room full of people. Yes, yes, you know there's nothing *really* to be afraid of—no one is going to boo, your skirt won't mysteriously fly up over your head, and no one will trip you on your way up to the microphone. It doesn't matter. As soon as your body gets wind of the fact that you intend to speak to a crowd, it kicks off its own agenda of anxiety. And it doesn't help one bit to know that your job depends on you doing a good job.

> Reduce the effects of stress on your body, and promote your natural talkativeness.

Practicing your speech helps ease the mental discomfort—but it also takes time, which you may not have. You need a magic bullet. Something that can take the edge off your anxiety, reduce the effects of stress on your body, and promote your natural talkativeness. Blessedly, the good people of the Polynesian islands discovered just such a remedy thousands of years ago. It's kava kava, an herbal remedy derived from the root of the kava plant. Traditionally used by Pacific island natives to boost feelings of goodwill and encourage storytelling before ceremonies, kava kava is now available at your local health food store. While nothing can solve all of your problems, kava kava is uniquely suited to take the sting out of anxiety-producing events, of which public speaking ranks way up at the top of the list.

(There is some controversy about kava kava's safety, so use it only on occasions when you legitimately need it and please see the modifications for further guidelines on its safe usage.) ❁

Remedy:
Kava Kava

Ingredients:
One bottle of kava kava tincture, available
at the health food store
A small glass of water or juice

Time Needed:
Mere seconds to take the kava kava;
twenty to thirty minutes for it to kick in

Instructions:
◉ Squirt half a dropper of kava kava in a small glass of water. As with all herbs, the right amount for you will depend on your size, metabolism, and sensitivity. As a guideline, the suggested dosage is one to three milliliters of tincture no more than three times a day.

◉ Down the hatch.

Modifications:
◉ If you can, spend a few moments sitting quietly and tuning in to the sound of your breath before it's your turn to speak. Calmness breeds calmness, so give yourself a nice serene place from which to start.

◎ Some studies suggest that kava kava can be toxic to the liver when taken regularly. If you have liver problems, such as hepatitis or cirrhosis, kava kava is not for you. (See the entry on Anxiety before a Big Meeting for another remedy.)

◎ For the same reason, do not consume alcohol while taking kava kava.

◎ Also skip the kava kava if you are taking any antianxiety, antipsychotic, or anticonvulsant medications, as it may impede the effectiveness or increase the side effects.

◎ As with anything, take it in moderation. Do not allow yourself to become dependent upon it.

Benefits:

◎ Kava kava takes the edge off your anxiety, which will help prevent that telltale hitch in your voice that makes it sound as if you are about to pass out.

◎ This herbal remedy promotes feelings of well-being, allowing your winning personality to shine through your presentation.

◎ Finally, it boosts communication skills. And honestly, is there anything more vital to being a good speaker?

Other Remedies to Try:
Alternate Nostril Breathing
Eyebrow Massage • Head Down Time Out
Swim in Your Own Sea of Tranquility

Asking for a Raise

he time has come for you to ask for more money, maybe even a promotion. No matter how much you feel you deserve it, it's still an emotional moment; you're asking your employer to recognize your worth. You're also opening yourself up to the possibility of rejection, which is always nerve-racking. And you need to strike just the right balance of conviction and humility, all while keeping your hands from shaking and your voice from quaking.

First, remember that asking for what you need makes you much more likely to receive it. No matter what happens in that meeting, you'll acquire extremely valuable practice in voting for yourself. Remember, too, that you need to remain open to hearing what your boss has to say, good and bad, so that if the answer is "no," you'll know exactly what you need to do to make the answer "yes" the next time. To achieve all of these aims, you need a combination of confidence, fortitude, and receptivity. This remedy can help you cultivate these traits and give you something to do in those moments before your meeting when the jitters are most likely to strike. Do the full pose in the privacy of your own home before you leave for work in the morning. Then take forty-five seconds to refresh your memory of the experience with an abbreviated version right before your meeting. You know how much you deserve this raise—now go in there and show 'em you're worth it. 🌸

Remedy:
Warrior 2 Pose

Ingredients:
At home: Shoeless feet and loose clothing
At work: Just a little privacy

Time Needed:
Two minutes at home in the morning
plus forty-five seconds at your desk or in an empty
conference room right before your meeting

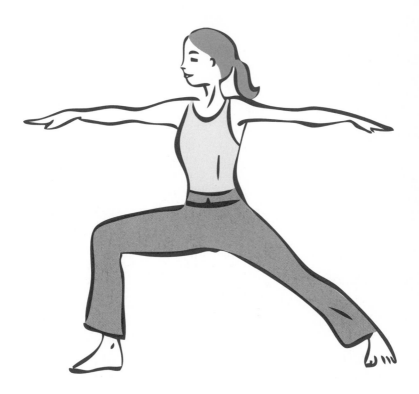

Instructions:

At home:

◎ Stand with your bare feet together and your hands on your hips.

◎ Stretch your arms out to your sides at shoulder height and extend your fingers.

◎ Move your feet apart so that your ankles are in line with your wrists.

◎ Turn your right toes 90 degrees to the right, and turn your left toes in 30 degrees.

◎ Reach down through your feet and out through your fingertips to get energy coursing throughout your body.

◎ Relax and broaden your chest and abdomen.

◎ Bend your right knee until your right thigh becomes as close to parallel to the floor as you can get.

◎ Turn your head to the right and gaze out over your right fingertips.

◎ Stay here and breathe five deep breaths. Feel the strength in your legs and arms and the softness in your belly and chest.

◎ After five breaths, straighten both legs and bring your hands to your hips to rest for a moment.

◎ Reverse the direction of your feet, re-extend your arms, and come into the pose on the left side. Stay another five breaths.

At work, remind yourself of the power you cultivated this morning by doing this mini version of the pose:

◎ Sit in your desk chair with both feet planted firmly on the ground. Your hips should remain pointing straight ahead of you.

◎ Extend your arms out to your sides at shoulder height.

🌀 Rotate your torso and your neck to look out over your right fingertips. Hold for two deep breaths.

🌀 Now reverse directions and look out over your left fingertips for two breaths.

Modifications:

🌀 The full pose requires a lot of stamina. If after one or two breaths you start quivering or panting for breath, decrease the intensity. Either don't bend your leg so deeply, or keep your hands on your hips. Focus instead on keeping your spine tall, your legs energized, and your torso open.

Benefits:

🌀 Builds strength in the legs and makes you aware of your own power

🌀 Helps you feel your connection to the ground beneath your feet, which is calming and energizing

🌀 Opens the hips, abdomen, lungs, and heart, allowing you to see how it is possible to be vulnerable and strong at the same time

🌀 Cultivates focus (As you gaze out over your fingertips, you practice setting your sights on a goal and not letting anything knock you off base.)

Other Remedies to Try:
Center of Power Stimulation • Get Grounded

Fight with Boss, Coworker, or Client

Perhaps your coworker copied your boss on a snippy e-mail. Or your boss took credit for one of your ideas. Or a particularly needy client finally made one demand too many. Whatever happened, you're seething. The challenge is to stand up for yourself while still maintaining your professionalism, which means screaming, snarling, or pitching any kind of fit are all out of the question.

It may take every ounce of reserve that you have, but the best thing you can do when a tide of anger threatens to overwhelm you is to remove yourself from the situation. You don't have to excuse yourself for the rest of the day, just long enough to regain your composure. And with a little help from this exercise, you can experience the release you're craving in mere seconds. You simply need somewhere private to do it. (This may seem like a tall order, but even Superman needed a minute to himself in a phone booth every once in a while.) Think of it as an instant catharsis. Once you've had a chance to expel some of that visceral anger, you'll be much more able to respond to the situation with calmness and clarity.

Think of it as an instant catharsis.

Remedy:
Lion Pose in the Bathroom

Ingredients:
Privacy

Time Needed:
Thirty seconds

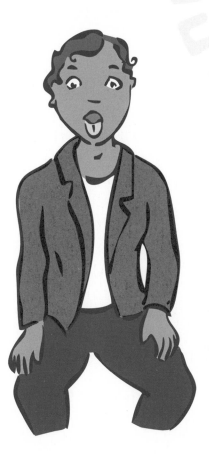

Instructions:

Sit up tall on the, ahem, toilet. Hey, you've got to work with what you've got—if the bathroom is your only choice, so be it. If you can, put the lid down so that you have a more secure seat.

◎ Rest your palms on your thighs.

◎ With your mouth closed, inhale deeply through your nose.

◎ As you exhale, stick your tongue out and open your eyes as wide as you can. Let your breath be forceful, as if you were a lion emitting a silent roar. Really let it rip and feel all the pent-up emotion draining from your body as you do.

◎ Repeat as necessary.

◎ When you feel purged, calmly walk back to your desk and *then* respond to the offending party.

Modifications:

◎ You can do this pose anywhere that's private—your car, a stairwell, your office (if you have one), or an empty conference room.

Benefits:

◎ Purges tension from the face, jaw, neck, and chest

◎ Gives you an emotional outlet that doesn't require screaming at another person and further escalating the situation

◎ Stimulates the throat chakra, which helps you communicate your needs and hear the needs of others

Other Remedies to Try:
Chamomile Tea
Mini Loving Kindness Meditation
Tighten and Release

Computer Crashes

After checking your e-mail, your bank account, and the status of your eBay auctions, you finally settle down into a nice work groove. After a couple of hours of honest work, you're poised to complete your presentation for your lunch meeting. You're feeling pretty good about yourself. So good, in fact, that you decide to take a trip over to iTunes to download a high-energy song to listen to while putting the finishing touches on your PowerPoint, when . . . kablooey. You get the blue screen of death.

You push buttons frantically, trying to remember how long ago you last saved your work, while your heart rate soars, your breath becomes raspy, and your shoulders crawl up toward your ears.

Computer crashes can send even the most placid soul into a spiral of stress. While your data may or may not be lost, you don't have to completely wig out here. You have two powerful tools on your side: your breath and gravity. Taking one or two short minutes to breathe deeply and stretch your back will help you pull it together and not burst a blood vessel while you wait for the help desk to answer your call.

Remedy:
Chair Forward Bend

Ingredients:
Desk chair
Help desk, or a handy friend

Time Needed:
One to two minutes

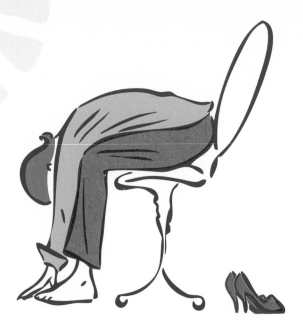

Instructions:

- It may take every ounce of your resolve, but move away from the keyboard and—literally—give yourself room to breathe. Push your chair back so that you have at least two feet of clearance between you and the desk.

- Scooch way back in the chair so that your spine touches the back rest.

- Separate your legs by bringing your knees to the outer edges of the chair seat.

- Take a deep breath while you lift the top of your head as far as you can toward the ceiling.

- As you exhale, bend forward at your hips, lay your torso on the inside of your thighs, and let your head and arms dangle toward the floor.

◎ Take ten deep breaths. Yes, ten. It will probably take you a full minute.

◎ As you inhale, try to feel your rib cage expanding in all directions. When you exhale, let your belly button rise in and up toward your spine.

◎ Continue to let your head feel heavy. It weighs approximately ten pounds—about the weight of a bowling ball. And since you purchased this book and are obviously smarter than the average soul, your head likely weighs more. Use the weight of your massive brain to draw your spine longer and longer.

◎ After your ten breaths (or longer, if it's feeling good), roll up in slow motion, stacking your lower back on top of your pelvis, your middle back on top of your lower back, and your upper back on top of your middle back. Bring your head up last.

◎ Now calmly call the help desk, or your most tech-savvy friend. (And best of luck.)

Modifications:

◎ If you're at work and someone asks you what you're doing, just tell them you dropped your pen. When they see the serene look on your face when you're done, they may just want to try a chair forward bend for themselves.

◎ If ten breaths feel so eternal that you start to get impatient, by all means, stay for a shorter period of time. Aim for five breaths instead. You can't let your stress remedy stress you out.

Benefits:

⊚ Getting your head lower than your heart helps your brain chill out so that you can keep this minor—albeit incredibly annoying—setback in perspective.

⊚ The slow, deep breaths trigger your body's relaxation response—your heart rate slows, your adrenal glands stop pumping out the adrenaline, and your nervous system calms down.

⊚ Your entire spine gets a big stretch, and your hips open, too, keeping your body supple and open despite the stress.

⊚ Think of successful athletes; they can hold it together during a clutch play. You're giving your body what it needs to keep you sharp. And you're gonna need it since you now have thirty minutes to re-create an entire presentation. Now go forth and conquer!

Other Remedies to Try:
Eyebrow Massage • Seated Spinal Twist

Anxiety before a Big Meeting

Perhaps you're kicking off a major project, presenting to a new client, or pitching an idea to your boss. Whatever the case, you have a big meeting where the stakes are decidedly higher than your usual doodle-in-your-note-book-to-keep-from-dozing-off meeting. You need to find something to occupy you while you wait, and you need a release valve for the mounting tension.

> *You need a release valve for the mounting tension.*

This self-massage technique used in Ayurveda, the school of traditional Indian medicine, is deceptively simple. It gives you something to do with your hands, ushers tension out of the body, and helps take your mind off your worries. Best of all, you can do it surreptitiously while seated at your desk.

Remedy:
Eyebrow Massage

Ingredients:
A desk and a chair

Time Needed:
One to two minutes

Instructions:

- Sit in your chair close to your desk.

- Rest your elbows on the desk.

- Lean your head forward so that you can bring your thumbs to the inner corners of both eyebrows.

🌀 Let the weight of your head sink into your thumbs for a few moments.

🌀 Now gently but firmly pinch the skin of your eyebrows between your thumbs and index fingers. Hold for one second, then move your hands out slightly and repeat.

🌀 Work your way to the outer edges of your eyebrows.

🌀 Repeat two or three times.

🌀 When you're done, slowly lift your head back up to vertical and notice any difference you feel.

Modifications:

🌀 If you feel really tense, you may experience some mild muscle soreness. This is normal and simply a sign that you were truly in need.

Benefits:

🌀 Releases stored tension in the face from when you wrinkle your brow

🌀 Calms your thoughts (Dropping your head forward sends a signal to your brain to cool it.)

🌀 Eases headaches

🌀 Brightens your outlook (It may be subtle, but when you lift your head after this exercise, you'll feel just a little lighter mentally than before you began.)

🌀 Gives you something to do with your hands while you're waiting for the appointed time to arrive

Other Remedies to Try:
Chamomile Tea • Head Down Time Out
Swim in Your Own Sea of Tranquility

Afternoon Slump

The three o'clock hour is a dangerous time of day: Lunch is well behind you, quitting time is still hours away, and you're getting so sleepy that your keyboard is starting to look like a pillow. It's a common impulse to reach for an afternoon hit of sugar or caffeine, or both, to give you the little lift you need to sail through the rest of the work day. But a sweet treat or a Venti double latte will only leave you feeling more depleted when their manufactured highs wear off. To top it off, they are also highly caloric with little nutritional value to show for it. Plus, they can be an expensive daily habit!

Get your energy humming again without even getting out of your chair.

Luckily, your body is equipped with an inherent supply of energy. The trick is to build it up, not drain it. According to Chinese medicine, the kidneys are the body's primary manufacturers of the vital energy known as *qi* (pronounced "chee"). By taking two minutes to complete this move, which stimulates an important point along the kidney meridian (or pathway of energy), you can get your energy humming again without even getting out of your chair. You may still decide to have a cookie or a coffee drink, but you'll know that you're opting to have it because you want it, not because you need it. And somehow, that makes it taste even a little sweeter. ❀

Remedy:
Office Chair Twist

Ingredients:
An office chair that swivels
A desk

Time Needed:
Two minutes

Instructions:

- Hold on to the edge of your desk with both hands.

- Push yourself and your chair straight back away from the desk until your arms are almost straight.

- Pick your feet up off the floor.

- Keeping your knees bent, and using your hands as leverage, swivel to your right until your knees are parallel to the edge of your desk. Your shoulders remain pointing straight toward your desk.

- Now use your hands to smoothly swivel to the left.

- Keep going, flowing back and forth and breathing rhythmically as you do, for two minutes.

- Concentrate on feeling stimulated and energized in the area of your back just beneath the clasp of your bra.

Modifications:

🌀 Because this twist also affects the digestive system, wait two hours after a big meal before doing it so that you don't interrupt the digestive process.

🌀 If you don't have an office chair that swivels, see the remedy for Lethargy—a simple standing exercise that stimulates the same region of the spine and has a similarly energizing effect. You will have to find a mostly uncluttered (and likely private) room to do it in.

Benefits:

🌀 Stimulates the kidneys, the body's main source of vital energy according to Chinese medicine

🌀 Gently twists the spine, which promotes flexibility, reduces stress, and promotes digestion and detoxification

🌀 Boosts your fun quotient for the afternoon—how long has it been since you last played with your office chair?

🌀 Proves that not every self-care routine has to be meditative and serious

🌀 Helps you become aware of your breath, which paves the way for you to breathe more deeply, which helps you relax

---

Other Remedies to Try:
Hot Ginger Tea • Powerful Breath
Ring the Gong • Seated Spinal Twist

Transitioning Out of Work Mode

You've been sitting all day. Your legs have been totally under-utilized and are borderline numb. But your back is full of sensation; it's aching from the effort of keeping you upright and motionless for hours at a time. It's no way to embark on the good part of life—your free time. You don't want to feel so wiped out from work that you can't enjoy your evening.

> You don't want to feel so wiped out from work that you can't enjoy your evening.

Creating a ritual that eases the transition between employee and normal person can help you leave stress at the office and make the most of your evenings and week-ends. And choosing a ritual that's ridiculously easy, incredibly short, and totally indulgent will help ensure that you actually do it with some regularity. Here's a suggestion to help you transition with grace.

Remedy:
Standing Forward Bend

Ingredients:
Shoeless feet
A modicum of privacy—if you're worried about getting strange looks from your coworkers, it might be best to save this for when you get home

Time Needed:
Two minutes

Instructions:

◉ Stand with your feet (shoeless, so you don't get thrown off balance by any kind of high heel) one fist's distance apart and your hands on your hips. You want the outer edges of your feet to be parallel to one another; take a moment to check that your toes aren't pointing in or out.

◉ Reach down through your feet and up through the back of your neck to make your body as tall as it can be.

◉ Gently engage your thigh muscles. If you have no idea how to do this, try lifting your kneecaps by squeezing the fronts of your thighs. You don't want to grip really tightly; you just want to energize the quadriceps (the muscles in the fronts of your thighs) to keep you stable and allow your hamstrings (the backs of your thighs) to gently release.

◉ Fold forward at the hips and bring your torso down as far as it can comfortably go over your legs. You'll be looking at your knees or thighs.

◉ Release your head. Let it be heavy.

◉ Let your arms dangle down toward the floor and rest wherever they can comfortably reach—on the floor, the tops of your feet, the outside of your ankles, your shins, or your thighs.

◉ Keep all effort contained to your lower body while your entire upper body grows softer, longer, and more relaxed.

◉ Stay here and breathe deeply for five to ten breaths. Feel your spine gradually unwind to bring you farther down over your legs as you do.

◎ To come up, bring your hands back to your hips, bend your knees slightly, and slowly roll up one vertebra at a time. Let your head be the last thing to arrive.

Modifications:

◎ If your hamstrings are screaming at you because the stretch is too intense, bend your knees until the sensation is tolerable.

◎ If you just don't come over very far, rest your palms on your thighs and concentrate instead on extending the spine long and parallel to the floor. Look forward so that your lifted chin also stretches the top of your chest and front of your neck.

Benefits:

◎ Stretches and strengthens the legs, waking them up from their long day's nap

◎ Releases tension from the spine, which has been over-working (kind of like you)

◎ Rejuvenates the entire body so that you can enjoy your time off

◎ Quiets the mind so that you can leave whatever happened at work today at work

Other Remedies to Try:
Shoulder Bounces
Stimulate Your "Letting Go" Acupressure Point

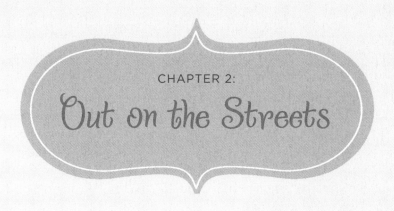

CHAPTER 2:

Out on the Streets

The rules of decorum are a little looser when you're out mingling with the public than when you're on the job. You aren't required to act as a representative of any entity other than yourself, and if something irritates you, there are no rules against raising your voice or honking your horn. But you still want to maintain a modicum of composure. First, you don't want to ruin your mood by allowing the inevitable annoyance to get you all riled up. And you certainly don't want to wind up on YouTube, caught on a camera phone in a shouting match with a bus driver. Here are some simple ways to keep your cool that you can do in a crowd without looking like a weirdo. May they help you get from point A to point B with your sanity and inherent good nature firmly intact.

Here are some simple ways to keep your cool that you can do in a crowd without looking like a weirdo.

Crowded Bus, Subway, Train

here are people filling every crevice of available space around you. You may even be forced to stand for what could be a long ride. You need something to help you settle in and enjoy the trip without getting so zoned out that you miss your stop. And because there are strangers on all sides of you, the remedy has to be inconspicuous and can't involve too much space.

> *This meditation technique takes place somewhere vast yet invisible—your mind.*

This meditation technique takes place somewhere vast yet invisible—your mind. You can keep doing it for however long it takes for you to reach your destination, and it will help you relax without dozing off. It's a listening meditation that requires you to think like a tape recorder.

As humans, we tend to listen to something by zeroing in on whatever we want to hear and turning down our awareness of any background noise. But tape recorders don't discriminate between noises; they record whatever travels through the microphone. In this exercise, you want to use your brain like a tape recorder and concentrate on hearing everything there is to hear without allowing your attention to get drawn to one particular sound. It's yet another way to give your mind something to focus on so that it can stop spinning on the hamster wheel of your everyday thoughts. Even though it requires concentration, it gives your mind a rest. And where the mind goes, the body follows (and vice versa).

Remedy:
The Human Tape Recorder

Ingredients:
Attention and intention

Time Needed:
As long as you remain in your crowded space

Instructions:

◎ Sit or stand up tall.

◎ Turn your attention to focus on what you can hear. You'll likely notice that one noise jumps out at you, and it's probably the loudest or most annoying.

◎ Now see what else you can hear at the same time. Try to divide your attention equally between every noise that enters your ears. It can be hard to do at first, but it does become easier with practice. It's also fairly mind-blowing to discover how many things you normally tune out.

◎ Notice when a particular sound has drawn your full attention or when you've drifted off into a daydream, and resume dividing your focus between everything you can hear.

◎ You decide how long to keep it up, whether it's until you reach your destination, or when you've become noticeably calmer. Before you immerse yourself back in your normal thoughts, however, note how you feel differently than you did when you started. It may be a subtle or profound difference—either way is perfect.

Modifications:

◎ You can do this with eyes open or closed. Although eyes open may be less noticeable to your fellow passengers (and safer when taking public transportation), it's generally easier to concentrate with your eyes closed.

◎ Be careful not to veer into blatant eavesdropping. Although it may be tempting, and you will likely overhear snippets of highly entertaining conversation, the point of this exercise isn't to invade others' privacy. It's to cultivate your own peace of mind. So when you hear some juicy revelation, note it and move on.

◎ Be sure to try this technique the next time you are out in nature. If doing it on a crowded train is interesting, imagine the beautiful sounds you'll be able to hear in the great outdoors.

Benefits:

◎ Quiets your thoughts, which is relaxing to both mind and body

◎ Helps hone your powers of awareness

◎ Turns a normally stressful and unavoidable part of your day into an opportunity to clear your mental slate and emerge refreshed

◎ Helps you wake up to the intricacy of every single moment

Other Remedies to Try:
4-7-8 Breath
People Watching as Spiritual Exercise
Slow Breath

Dealing with Aggressive People

Some people—drunk guys in bars, impatient line-waiters, and taxi stealers—just don't take no for an answer. When confronted with someone hell-bent on getting something from you, even if it's simply your attention, it's easy to become flustered. You hope to hold your ground without escalating the situation and then take your (oh so graceful) leave, but often, some part of you just wants to crawl under the nearest chair.

The key is to remember your own strength and to project it out into the world, showing your antagonist that you're no pushover. The problem is that as women we're often taught, consciously or subconsciously, that taking up as little space as possible makes us nice and desirable. In this instance, your best antidote is to inflate yourself through some simple postural adjustments. If your body projects confidence, your mind will follow suit. Whether we're aware of it or not, we're all projecting signals with our body language, and we're reading the signals of others. With this exercise, you'll broadcast the message "I'm powerful and I want you to back off, bub." Prepare to strike awe into the hearts of man. Or at least, hesitation. ❧

> *The key is to remember your own strength and to project it out into the world.*

Remedy:
Inflate Yourself

Ingredients:
The mental wherewithal to remember what to do in the heat of the moment

Time Needed:
As long as you need

Instructions:

◉ Start with your posture: Plant your feet flat on the ground and lift the back of your neck up toward the ceiling to unfurl to your full height. Keep your chin slightly lifted and your chest open. Voila—you instantly project more of a confident presence.

◉ Keep your hands by your sides or clasped behind your back. Crossing your arms in front of you blocks your abdomen. Why do you want to keep your belly exposed? Nearly every mind/body tradition, from yoga to *qigong* to martial arts, considers this area to be the source of your personal power. You don't want to hide it.

◉ Keep your knees soft to go with the flow but reach down into the floor through the soles of your feet to draw strength from a solid sense of being grounded.

Modifications:

◉ Don't be afraid to make noise and draw the attention of those around you if you need back up. Hollering, whistling, clapping your hands, or banging your hands on anything nearby all work.

Benefits:

◉ Enables you to take some control of a situation in which the other person has monopolized that control

◎ Allows you to access your inner—and sometimes hidden—
stores of confidence

◎ Literally teaches you to "stand up for yourself"

Other Remedies to Try:
Complete Breath • Goddess Pose

Stuck in Traffic

You're going nowhere fast. As you watch the minutes creep by and your gas tank inch lower and lower, you can feel your tension level rise as your shoulders inch up toward your ears. On top of it all, you must remain somewhat alert—no zoning out allowed. If only you could sip a margarita while you sit. Dang those open container laws!

This simple movement releases stress while it reinvigorates you so you'll have more energy available to pay attention. Best of all, it's an easy way to build a little more fun into your day. And who doesn't need that? ✿

Remedy:
Shoulder Bounces

Ingredients:
A willingness to look a little funny and
a sincere desire to release tension
Good music

Time Needed:

Until traffic starts flowing again

Instructions:

- Sit up tall in your seat.

- Rest your hands on the top of your steering wheel so your shoulders are more or less even (one isn't higher than the other).

- Start by slowly lifting your shoulders up to your ears and letting them drop back down.

- Gradually pick up the speed of your bounces until you get a comfortable rhythm.

- With each bounce, imagine you're literally shaking stress off your body.

- Stop when you get tired and start again when you find that tension creeping back in.

Modifications:

- Crank the radio—it helps unlock those frozen shoulders and makes the whole enterprise a little more fun.

- If the bounces feel too monotonous, move your torso in any way that feels cathartic to you. Just be sure to keep the majority of your attention on the road!

Benefits:

- Loosens up that chronically tight shoulder/neck area

- Invites a little enjoyment into an otherwise sucky part of your day

◉ Teaches that movement doesn't have to be structured or complicated to have an effect on your state of mind

Other Remedies to Try:
4-7-8 Breath • Lion Pose in the Bathroom
Swim in Your Own Sea of Tranquility
Tighten and Release

Road Rage

Whether someone cut you off, honked at you, or tailed a little too closely, some relatively minor driving transgression has elicited a whopper of a response from you. There's something about being sealed inside your own pod of a car that makes it feel safe to really let your anger fly. After all, they can't hear what you're saying. Why not curse them, their mother, their dog, and all future generations of their offspring? No one will ever know, right?

It's kind of like the age-old question: If a tree falls in the woods, and there's no one around to hear it, does it make a noise? Really, it doesn't matter if there was a noise or not. The tree still fell. If you launch into a violent rant that no one can hear, you still give anger a green light to overtake your body and influence your actions.

Just because you're choosing not to act out of anger, however, doesn't mean you need to swallow it or pretend it doesn't exist. You simply need a way to consciously release it. This exercise helps you acknowledge that you are experiencing a surge of ire, and then issues an invitation for your anger to dissipate. You will feel so much better if you do this than if you yell and honk and get all red in the face, because you'll be purging tension instead of escalating it. Let the catharsis begin! ❦

Remedy:
Tighten and Release

Ingredients:
Just enough awareness to realize that you are about to fly off the handle
The focus to choose a more conscious reaction

Time Needed:
One to two minutes

Instructions:

◉ Take one or two deep breaths to set the stage.

◉ Start at the top of your body and work your way down. Inhale and squeeze your face (while still keeping your eyes on the road, of course) as tight as you can, and then release all that effort with an exhale.

◉ Draw your shoulders up toward your ears and hold them there for a beat, then exhale and let them drop back down.

◉ Squeeze the steering wheel as tightly as you can and tighten all the muscles in your arms, then release.

◉ Pull your belly button in as strongly as you can, hold for a moment, then let that effort go.

◎ Clench your butt, thighs, calves, and your feet (again, only go as far as feels safe, or wait until you're at a red light) as tightly as you can and then exhale and release.

◎ Once you've swept your whole body, repeat the process another time or two. Each time you do, you'll root out more tension.

Modifications:

◎ You can use this technique anytime someone trips your anger wires. It can be done on a brisk walk around the block, at your desk, or even on a crowded flight.

Benefits:

◎ Targets the entire body and systematically releases tension from every corner

◎ Gives you a practical way to soothe yourself, instead of just thinking, "I need to relax"

◎ Helps you refrain from escalating the situation or laying on the horn and spreading your aggression to everyone within earshot of your car

Other Remedies to Try:
Lion Pose in the Bathroom
Mini Loving Kindness Meditation
Shoulder Bounces

Running Late

Maybe you dropped the ball and overslept, or maybe something completely out of your control popped up to throw a wrench in your schedule. Either way, you really need to be somewhere five minutes ago, and there is nothing you can do to accelerate your travel time. Before you even walk out the door, your stress levels are spiking. And then on every step of your journey—walking to the car or public transportation, driving or riding, parking, walking the final few steps to your ultimate destination—they keep on climbing.

Running late also creates the opportunity for your own self-importance to spiral out of control. If someone is walking or driving too slowly in front of you, all you can think is, "Out of my way! Can't you see I'm late?!" Which basically translates as, "I am more important than you." Ew.

You need a way to get grounded and you must be able to do it even while you're moving as quickly as possible. This meditation technique offers the chill pill you so desperately need as it takes focus off the drama created by your lateness. Best of all, it's portable and can travel wherever you need to go.

Remedy:
Count Your Breaths

Ingredients:
Attention

Time Needed:
At least one full minute for a noticeable effect (but you can keep it up until you reach your destination)

Instructions:

◎ As you walk, drive, or ride, count each exhale. You can do it silently or audibly, whichever works best for you.

◎ When you get to ten, start again at one.

◎ Keep going until you're breathing a little more deeply and your mind is churning a little more slowly. (And you don't want to knock over anyone who's moving too slowly ahead of you.)

Modifications:

◎ When you find that you've lost track, or that you've reached eighteen without realizing it, start again. No beating yourself up allowed. Everyone's mind will wander. The only crucial step is noticing that you've gotten off track and then getting back to it.

Benefits:

◎ Takes the focus off exactly how late you are

◎ Gives your mind a chance to rest and helps to quiet your entire nervous system

◎ Promotes a relaxed awareness, which you'll need when you finally reach your destination

> **Other Remedies to Try:**
> Stress Scan • Tighten and Release

Lost

ou're cruising along on your way, when suddenly you realize nothing looks familiar. Crud! You've gone and gotten lost. Not knowing where you are is a pretty emotionally unstable place to be. Plus, this little detour probably means that you're now going to be late. Cue the anxiety! (And don't forget to read the previous entry on Running Late.)

Of course, there is another way—one that doesn't require a global positioning device or an iPhone. You can take action to ground yourself before you completely spin out of control, lose the ability to think rationally, and get yourself lost even further.

> You can take action to ground yourself before you completely spin out of control.

Acupressure is essentially acupuncture that you perform on yourself by applying pressure to specific points on your body—no needles required. According to traditional Chinese medicine (TCM), we are filled with vital energy, or *qi* (pronounced "chee"), that flows through the body along pathways known as meridians. Certain points on these meridians are associated with specific mental and physical functions. Stimulating these points with focused pressure encourages *qi* to flow through them, which in turn brings balance to the point itself as well as the mental and physical functions that the point regulates. TCM teaches that the point in the center of your breastbone, known as the Sea of Tranquility, reduces anxiety, nervousness, and panic. Stimulating the Sea of Tranquility helps you find a feeling of stillness when your surroundings are whirling. ❁

Remedy:
Swim in Your Own Sea of Tranquility

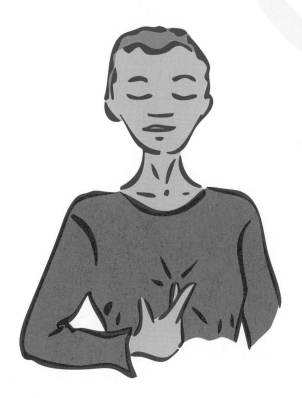

Ingredients:

One middle finger

Time Needed:

Two minutes

Instructions:

🌀 To find your Sea of Tranquility, locate the small indentation that's approximately the width of three fingers from the bottom of your breastbone—generally just above nipple height in the space between your boobs. (It may sound like this would be awkward to find in public, but you can pretend you're merely scratching an itch and no one will be the wiser.)

🌀 Press the tip of one of your middle fingers into the Sea of Tranquility. Start with gentle pressure, and gradually increase to a moderate intensity. You don't need to bore a hole in your chest! You merely need to bring attention to the area.

🌀 Close your eyes if you can and breathe slowly, easily, and fully into the space beneath your fingertip. Aim to take twenty breaths, which should take about two minutes.

🌀 Release the pressure gradually, and take a few breaths at the very end with only a light touch.

Modifications:

🌀 For the love of Pete, ask for directions when you're done.

Benefits:

🌀 Opens the chest and invites your breath to deepen, which triggers the body's relaxation response

🌀 Helps regulate your heartbeat, so you don't have that pounding-in-your-chest feeling adding to your stress levels

🌀 Calms the mind as well as the body, so you can think clearly enough to get back on track

Other Remedies to Try:
4-7-8 Breath • Count Your Breaths
Stress Scan

Motion Sickness

You like planes, trains, automobiles, and boats, but they don't like you. There's nothing like a little jostling to get you green around the gills. There's also an emotional component that feeds the physical nausea. Have you ever noticed that you rarely get motion sickness when you're driving, but when you're stuck in the middle of the backseat, you start feeling sick? It's called not being in control—a concept that can be deeply unsettling, particularly when you're not standing on solid ground. It's enough to turn your stomach.

Once again, acupressure comes to the rescue. There's a spot on your inner forearm called the Inner Gate—the same point that "motion sickness bands" are designed to stimulate—that has the power to combat stomach upset and nausea. It also has the added benefit of easing anxiety. A few minutes of gentle pressure and deep breathing and you should be ready to go with the flow. ✿

Remedy:
Open Your Inner Gate

Ingredients:
Time
Breath
Two hands

Time Needed:
Four minutes

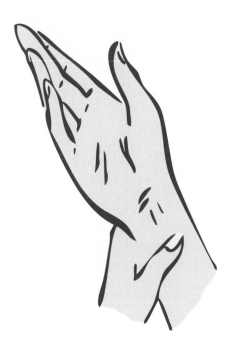

Instructions:

🌀 Find the Inner Gate on your left inner arm—it's two-and-a-half finger widths up from the crease where your forearm meets the bottom of your hand.

🌀 Place your right thumb on this spot and wrap your fingers around the other side of your forearm.

🌀 Apply gentle but constant pressure with your thumb while you take ten to twelve deep breaths—about one minute.

◎ After one minute move your thumb one-half finger width closer to your wrist crease and press there for another minute.

◎ Repeat on your right arm.

Modifications:

◎ This point can also be used to ease insomnia caused by emotional upset.

Benefits:

◎ Makes you an active participant in your quest to feel better, which helps give you back some sense of control

◎ Gives you something to focus on other than how crappy you're feeling

◎ Soothes a churning stomach

◎ Calms the mind and lessens anxiety

Other Remedies to Try:
Complete Breath • Hot Ginger Tea

Waiting

The sun is shining and people are walking down the street, going wherever they please, but not you. No. You are stuck in the mother of all lines at the post office, sitting in the waiting room at the doctor's office, or wondering if they will ever call you for jury duty. No matter where you are, your life has come to a screeching halt and you have very little information about how long it will be until your wait is over. You can huff and puff and hop from one foot to the other all you want, but nothing you do will expedite the process.

Being forced to wait has an uncanny ability to make you feel trapped. It is nature's way of reminding you that while you may be able to travel halfway around the world in a matter of hours, you're still not in complete control of your life. At some point, you're going to have to stand or sit in one spot and wait until someone else tells you it's your turn to get what you need.

You could use the imposed delay as an opportunity to stress out about all the things you need to do when you are finally free. Or you could rehash the events that happened earlier in the day. If those don't appeal, perhaps you could daydream about something that may never happen. But let's face it—none of these options is particularly helpful. So what's a bored girl to do?

You simply need to be still and notice what is happening in this precise moment.

Here's a simple way to keep yourself occupied that also helps you become a little less reactive to stressful situations. This exercise encourages you to cultivate mindfulness, which renowned Zen Buddhist teacher Thich Nhat Hanh defines as "keeping one's consciousness alive to the present reality," and what American guru Ram Dass is referring to when he says, "Be here now." When you practice mindfulness, you fully open yourself to the events in any given moment instead of spending your precious time fixated on something you're about to do or something that has already occurred. You simply need to be still and notice what is happening in this precise moment. And since you're not going anywhere any time soon, you already have the "sit still" part covered. As far as noticing is concerned, it gives you something fascinating on which to rest your attention—your fellow humans. Prepare to be riveted and feel more relaxed. ✿

Remedy:
People Watching as Spiritual Exercise

Ingredients:
Time
Attention

Time Needed:
As long as you have to wait

Instructions:

◎ To set the stage for being aware and staying awake, place both feet on the floor and sit up tall in your chair. (If you're standing, be sure your weight is distributed evenly across the soles of both feet and lift the crown of your head up to stand up straight.)

◎ Place your hands in your lap or rest them on your armrests— no crossing them in front of your torso—to keep your body language open and receptive. You want to take in what's going on, not block it out. (If you're standing, hold your hands by your sides or clasp them behind your back.)

🌀 Begin looking around the room with the sole intention of seeing whatever there is to see.

🌀 Notice your surroundings. What immediately draws your attention? The biggest character in the room, or the quiet person over in the corner?

🌀 Your goal isn't to judge what you see, only to observe it. When you find your attention wandering, or your mind making judgments about what you see, begin again with your pure observation.

🌀 Although you want to refrain from forming opinions about what you observe, you don't have to remain completely stoic. You want to see what you see, notice your reaction to it, and then return to simply observing.

🌀 Keep going, and start again as many times as you need to.

Modifications:

🌀 You can choose to focus on one area, or take in everyone in the whole room at once. You can even alternate between the two at a leisurely pace to evenly work your nearsighted and farsighted people-watching muscles.

🌀 Whatever you choose, you don't want to stare so intently at someone that you make them uncomfortable. Keep your gaze gentle, as if what you were seeing were rising up to meet you instead of projecting your focus strongly out into the room.

Benefits:

🌀 Keeps you from thinking about all the things you aren't doing because you are stuck here, thereby reducing stress

@ Cultivates curiosity about your fellow humans, which is the precursor to compassion

@ Promotes awareness—how often are you this cognizant of everything that's going on around you?

@ Sets the stage for a formal meditation practice, since meditating is all about noticing your thoughts in the same way you were noticing the people around you—without judgment and with gentle concentration

@ Provides free—and endless—entertainment

Other Remedies to Try:
The Human Tape Recorder
Stimulate Your "Letting Go" Acupressure Point

Sitting on the Runway

Sitting on an airplane, waiting out a flight delay on the run-way, is perhaps the most frustrating of all "out on the street" predicaments, because you are forced to sit still—often, you can't even get up to go to the bathroom. You're literally trapped in a confined space as the minutes or hours slowly pass. You don't know how long you'll be there, or whether this means you'll miss your connecting flight or whatever you have planned for when you reach your destination. It's undeniably frustrating. And potentially claustrophobia-inducing. And beyond that, there are *so* many other things you could be doing. But for now, you must sit.

They may be able to force you to stay in your seat, but they can't keep you from doing a simple movement that will make you better able to swallow the delay without a lot of slumping and harrumphing. ❧

Remedy:
Seated Spinal Twist

Ingredients:
A willingness to do something outside the norm

Time Needed:
Two minutes—one minute for each side

Instructions:

◎ Place both feet flat on the floor, toes pointing straight ahead.

◎ Lift the back of your neck up so your spine lengthens and you sit up nice and tall.

◎ Rest your palms on the armrests.

◎ Inhale a big breath and grow as tall as you can.

◎ Exhale and use your hands as leverage to rotate your torso to the right.

◎ Stay for nine more breaths (for a total of ten), lifting the spine up with each inhale and gently rotating the torso farther to the right with each exhale.

◎ Come back to the center and take one or two normal breaths before repeating to the left side.

Modifications:

◎ You can turn your head in the direction of the twist (over your right shoulder, if you're twisting to the right), keep your head and gaze forward, or look over your left shoulder. Choose the option that feels most comfortable to your neck, and do the same thing when you twist to the other side.

◎ If you are self-conscious, remember that when your fellow passengers see how good this simple movement feels, they'll start secretly admiring you. Also keep in mind that it's really only the people in your row and the row directly behind you, and they're likely in need of distraction anyway.

Benefits:

◎ Wrings tension out of the muscles that support your spine, helping to prevent back pain

◎ Stimulates the abdominal organs responsible for digestion and detoxification so you don't get the upset stomach that often accompanies stress

◎ Promotes deeper breathing, which triggers relaxation

◎ Feels really good

Other Remedies to Try:
4-7-8 Breath
People Watching as Spiritual Exercise
Stimulate Your "Letting Go" Acupressure Point

Screaming Baby

While you know the baby is too young to know that it's not polite to shriek in public, its cry is so piercing it's making you want to jump out the window.

You can sit there and let every cry shave another layer off your nerves, or you can use it as an opportunity to practice becoming comfortable in an uncomfortable situation. Because, heaven knows, there's no avoiding uncomfortable situations—you may as well learn how to make the best of them.

> *This meditation technique can help you open your heart to anyone who's trying your patience.*

This meditation technique can help you open your heart to anyone who's trying your patience. Its aim is to cultivate something Tibetan Buddhists call *metta,* which translates to "loving kindness." Ultimately, this practice can help you feel warmly toward all people—even those who are otherwise driving you crazy or causing you pain. But for now, let's start with a helpless little baby who's having a hard time. Once you've got that down, you can build from there.

Remedy:
Mini Loving Kindness Meditation

Ingredients:
Attention

Time Needed:
A couple of minutes

Instructions:

◎ Sit up tall and place your feet flat on the floor.

◎ Start by turning your attention to your breathing for a few breaths. Concentrate on feeling the air flow in and out of your lungs.

◎ Once you're a little calmer, call up an image of the baby in your mind.

◎ Silently say to yourself, "May the baby be happy. May the baby be free from suffering." If this is too much of a mouthful for you or feels phony for any reason, try something simpler such as "Bless that baby's heart" (or a beneficent phrase of your own choosing).

◎ Whatever you decide to say, keep saying it. You can repeat it as slowly or as quickly as you like. What's important is that you find a rhythm that feels good to you.

◎ Try to feel the meaning of those words from the bottom of your heart—don't just robotically chant them.

◎ Continue for a minute or two; then return to simply focusing on your breath for a few moments.

Modifications:

◎ You can have your eyes open or closed, whatever feels best to you in your surroundings.

◎ You can also use this technique toward anyone who's trying your nerves. You might find it comes in handy after you've had a fight with someone you love, your mom drops by unannounced, or someone dings your car in the parking lot.

⊚ Perhaps the most important person you could direct your loving kindness to is yourself. Next time you make a mistake or a choice that negatively impacts your life, try taking two minutes to wish good things and an end of suffering for yourself. You are, after all, the most vital person in your life. You deserve the same good care you offer others.

Benefits:

⊚ A loving kindness meditation hones your ability to feel compassion. Instead of sitting there and hating that baby, you're sending it a little love. It's good for the baby and good for you.

⊚ This activity allows you to feel a connection to those around you (the baby, in this instance), instead of suffering in silence.

⊚ Meditation gives you something to focus on other than your irritation, which helps diminish your annoyance.

Other Remedies to Try:
4–7–8 Breath

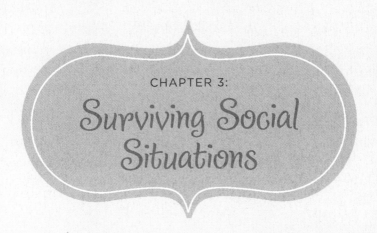

CHAPTER 3:
Surviving Social Situations

One of the many benefits of using natural remedies to deal with stressful situations is that the good effects extend beyond only you. When you're energized, relaxed, and feel you have some semblance of control over your reactions to life's little curve-balls, it not only improves your own well-being but also changes how you treat others. Think about how much better you can handle an awkward situation when you're well-rested and good-humored versus when you're tired, cranky, and out-of-sorts. And when you treat people more gently, they will in turn change how they act toward you. It's a beautiful chain reaction: You take better care of yourself>you feel better>you are nicer to other people>they in turn are nicer to you>you feel even better.

Commingling with your peers provides the perfect opportunity to test this magic theory, and it gives you a chance to build your treat-people-better muscles so that you can use them on your friends and family (which we'll get to in the next chapter). Try the following remedies when you are feeling socially challenged, and notice how they affect your actions and the actions of those around you.

First Date

You're going out tonight with a potential love interest, and you want to look and feel your best. But you don't want to go overboard, either—since it's too soon to tell if you'll be interested in scheduling a second date, you've decided to leave your sexiest stilettos in the closet (for now). You want to strike just the right balance between casualness and razzle-dazzle. You also need a way to calm your nerves and stay hopeful despite any skeptical voices in your head.

> *Strike just the right balance between casualness and razzle-dazzle.*

This easy facial massage comes to us from Ayurveda, the ancient school of medicine and self-care from India. According to Ayurveda, self-massage stimulates important energy points, helps to purge unwanted waste products, corrects any imbalances you may be experiencing, and promotes the rosy glow of well-being. Taking ten minutes to perform this facial massage can help you look your most radiant as you simultaneously release the stresses of your day—setting the stage perfectly for you to have a great time on your date.

Remedy:
Do-It-Yourself Face Massage

Ingredients:
An all-natural oil, such as sweet almond, sesame, or sunflower, available at your local health food store in the skin-care section
An essential oil that smells divine to you, such as lavender, rose, or geranium (optional)

Time Needed:
Ten minutes before showering

Instructions:
- Gently warm the all-natural oil by holding the bottle under hot running water for several seconds.

- Combine a small palmful of oil with three to five drops of your essential oil, if using, in a bowl.

- Dip the tips of your middle fingers into the oil, place them on the center of your chin, then rotate them clockwise for twenty to thirty seconds.

- Repeat for each of the following areas of your face: each corner of your mouth, the center of the indentation between your nose and upper lip, the outside edges of your nostrils, the very centers of your cheekbones, just beneath your eyes directly below your pupils, the inner edges of your eye socket just below the beginning of your eyebrows, your temples, and the spot directly in between your eyebrows. Replenish the oil on your fingertips before massaging each new spot.

- If you have time (and your skin is not super oily), rest for a few minutes and let the oil penetrate before getting in the shower. If not, proceed directly to the bath.

Modifications:
- If using the oil feels too greasy, you can skip it. Use your favorite moisturizer instead.

Benefits:

◎ Increases blood flow to the face, giving you a radiant glow

◎ Releases tension from your facial muscles, helping you look your most relaxed

◎ Allows you to direct a little attention and affection toward yourself, giving a boost to your overall sense of well-being

---

Other Remedies to Try:
Alternate Nostril Breathing
Arms Up, Chest Up

Attending an Event You Don't Want to Attend

You've been invited to a social function that sounds good in theory, but for some reason you can't seem to work up any enthusiasm about going. Maybe it's raining, or you won't know that many people there, or you're tired and some quality time with your couch and the remote control sounds so appealing right about now. But somewhere deep down you believe that you'll be glad you went if you can just get your butt out the door. You need fortitude and a burst of energy, and a good ol' standing yoga pose is the very thing to give it to you. Standing poses in general are energizing and grounding—which keeps you from over-thinking and rationalizing your way out of going.

Warrior 1 in particular opens the heart as it revitalizes the body, both of which help you be receptive to new experiences. Try it before you get in the shower to give you the oomph you need to get excited about the opportunities awaiting you. ❁

Remedy:
Warrior 1 Pose

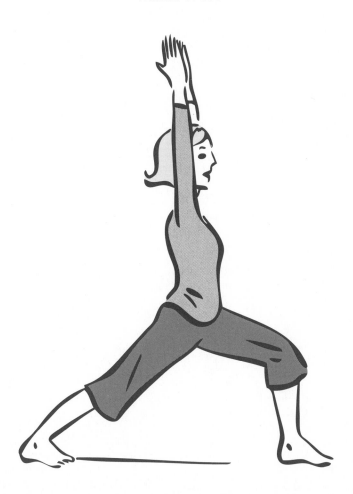

Ingredients:
Bare feet
Yoga mat (optional, although it does help
your feet feel more stable)
Nonrestrictive clothing

Time Needed:
Two minutes (thirty seconds for each side, twice)

Instructions:

- Start out standing with your big toes and heels touching, with your arms extending out to your sides at shoulder height.

- Step your feet about four feet apart. The space between your legs should roughly be equal to the length of one of your legs.

- Turn your right toes out 90 degrees to the right and your left toes in toward your right foot 30 degrees.

- Keeping your left heel firmly planted on the floor, turn your rib cage as far as you can to the right—ideally, your chest will face directly out over your right leg.

- Bend your right knee deeply so that your right shin is perpendicular to the floor.

- Lift your arms up alongside your ears and reach out through your fingertips. As you do this, take care to let your shoulder blades slide down your back so that there is space between your ears and the tops of your shoulders.

- Finally, lift up your rib cage and gently bend your upper spine back so you can reach up through your chest and turn your face to gaze steadily at your fingers.

◎ While in this pose, take five to ten breaths. Keep reaching back through your back heel, forward through your right shin, and up through your spine and fingers.

◎ Repeat to the left side.

◎ Rest for a few breaths with your feet together and hands on hips, then do the whole sequence one more time.

Modifications:

◎ If looking up at your hands makes you feel scrunched and tight in your shoulders, look straight ahead.

◎ The full pose requires you to bend your front leg so deeply that your thigh comes parallel to the floor. On your second pass, see if you can push yourself to drop a little more deeply into the pose.

◎ If keeping your back heel down or getting your chest to face forward is challenging, let that heel lift up so that you are on the ball of your back foot. Continue to reach that heel back to keep the leg strong.

Benefits:

◎ The physical challenge and steady gaze promote focus and stamina

◎ Strengthens the legs, shoulders, and back, making you a force to be reckoned with

◎ Opens the abdominal area, the seat of your personal power, and the chest, home of the heart, helping you find that magic combination of strength and receptivity

⊚ Releases tension from the hips and shoulders, helping you shed the stresses of the day so that you are more likely to have a fabulous time

> **Other Remedies to Try:**
> Arms Up, Chest Up • L-Shaped Handstand
> Legs Up the Wall

Going Out by Yourself

You have places to go—whether it's a party, wedding, bar, or restaurant—but you don't have the security blanket of having someone to walk in with. You *could* take a couple of tequila shots to get a dose of liquid courage, but then you might not make a great impression on the people you'll inevitably meet. (Plus, let's be realistic, you don't have the benefit of a designated driver). You're not going to allow that little pit of fear in your stomach prevent you from having a great time, are you?

Remember, you are much more likely to meet new people when you aren't surrounded by a gaggle of friends. Being alone makes you more approachable and more inclined to strike up conversations. You'll also be able to leave whenever you darn well please. And if you end up having a fantastic time, you won't have to head out simply because the person you came with is done for the night. To work up the gumption to go solo you need to purge the dread and remind yourself of your own fabulousness. You can do that by stimulating an acupressure point in your lower abdomen known as your Center of Power. ❀

Remedy:
Center of Power Stimulation

Ingredients:
Your two hands
A chair

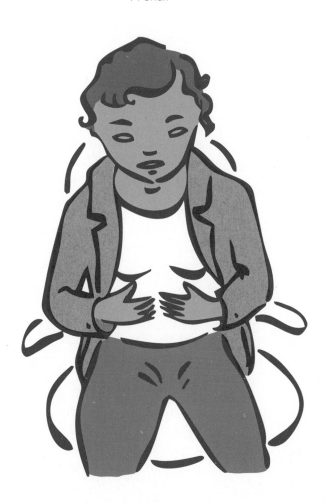

Time Needed:
A little over one minute

Instructions:

◉ Sit comfortably in your chair.

◉ Bring the tips of the fingers of both hands to your belly, equidistant between the bottom of your breastbone and your belly button. (The breastbone lies, aptly enough, between your boobs. To find where it ends, start just beneath the hollow in your throat, then trace a line straight down until the sensation beneath your fingers changes from hard to soft.)

◉ Slowly and steadily press your fingers in to your abdomen and slightly up.

◉ Lean your torso forward slightly to help you press more forcefully into your stomach.

◉ Breathe deeply for a full minute.

◉ Release the pressure slowly.

◉ Take a few normal breaths before jumping in to your night-out preparations.

Modifications/Cautions:

◉ Clearly, this won't feel too good if you've recently con-sumed a huge meal. Only do this exercise if you have a fairly empty stomach.

◉ Because this exercise uses deep pressure, it can be very stimulating, even over-stimulating if your health is vulner-able. Avoid this exercise if you have a chronic illness such as cancer, heart disease, or high blood pressure.

Benefits:

◎ Works to alleviate deep-seated insecurities that might otherwise keep you home

◎ Also good for relieving the upset stomach and tension headaches caused by stress and nervousness

◎ Ushers in new blood and energy to the abdomen, which is detoxifying and revitalizing for your digestive system as well as your perception of yourself

---

Other Remedies to Try:
Awkward Pose • Cobra Pose

Meeting People for the First Time

You're headed to a gathering—alone, or with others—where there will be lots of people you don't know. And while you're excited about the possibility of meeting folks who could become new friends, you're also a little intimidated—what if there's an awkward lull in conversation? What if everyone else there already knows one another? What if you get an attack of shyness and don't let your best self shine through?

Whenever you have to move past your comfort zone, it invites your insecurities to rise to the surface. The first step is to recognize your apprehension—after all, you can only change a habit that you're aware of having. Once you notice how you're feeling, you can take steps to move past your anxiety.

This exercise opens your chest and abdomen, mimicking that vulnerable feeling, and then encourages you to reach beyond your daily habits to make way for new breath, energy, and vitality to flow in. It's a great preparation for navigating those first few awkward moments and paving the way to having a great time. 🌸

> *Reach beyond your daily habits to make way for new breath, energy, and vitality to flow in.*

Remedy:
Arms Up, Chest Up

Ingredients:
Nonrestrictive clothing
Chair (optional)

Time Needed:
Two minutes

Instructions:

- You can sit or stand. If you're sitting, either sit on the edge of a hard chair or cross-legged on the floor.

- Interlace your fingers up to the webbing and straighten your arms out in front of you with your palms facing away from you.

- Exhale a breath here.

🌀 As you inhale, lift your arms above your head so that your palms are now facing the ceiling.

🌀 Reach through the palms to energize the muscles in your arms and to ensure that your elbows fully straighten.

🌀 Exhale and let your shoulders fall down away from your ears as your palms continue to reach up strongly.

🌀 Stay here and breathe deeply; feel the sides of your chest expand and your spine lengthen with each inhale. You want to feel that your torso is gradually growing bigger and taller as you remain in this pose. Aim for ten full breaths.

🌀 Bring your arms down on an exhale.

🌀 Rest for a moment, then change the interlace of your fingers so the opposite index finger is on top and repeat.

Modifications:

🌀 You can do this exercise in your parked car just before going into the party by crossing your forearms over each other, like *I Dream of Jeannie,* and lifting your bent arms over your head.

🌀 You can also do it any time you want to energize yourself, move past old thought patterns, and open yourself up to new experiences.

Benefits:

🌀 Encourages your breath to deepen, which simultaneously relaxes and revitalizes

🌀 Promotes focus and stamina (As your arms get tired, you will have to concentrate in order to stick with it for ten breaths.)

🌀 Creates space in the rib cage, the home of the heart, which helps you create more space in your metaphorical heart for new people

🌀 Counteracts depression, which often accompanies a sunken chest

🌀 Opens the shoulders and helps you reach past your perceived limits

> **Other Remedies to Try:**
> Alternate Nostril Breathing
> Kava Kava • Squat

Throwing a Party

The party is happening at your house tonight, and whether it's a casual get-together or a full-fledged soiree, you still want to look your best and have plenty of energy and attention to shower on your guests. The problem is you're running around like crazy making sure everything is tended to before folks arrive, and you're feeling scattered and slightly stressed.

Yes, you have a million things to do before your guests arrive. But before you hop in the shower, take sixty seconds to do this simple forward bend. Moving your head lower than your heart is called an inversion in yoga, and inversions are our friends for a variety of powerful reasons. First, lowering your head quiets the mind and gives your heart a chance to take the lead. It also increases circulation and, therefore, energy, by giving your heart a break from its normal patterns and allowing blood to flow effortlessly throughout the body. Finally, inversions reverse gravity—that pesky force responsible for the toll aging takes on our skin. Spending even ten deep breaths (which will take you about a minute) upside down will give you a subtle face-lifting effect, no botulism spores or needles required. ❃

Remedy:
Standing Wide-Legged Forward Bend

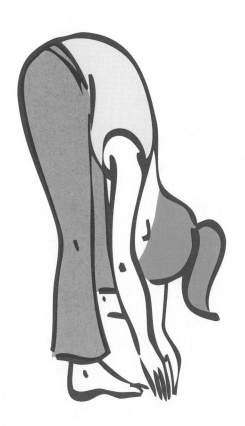

Ingredients:
Bare feet
Yoga mat or a non-slidy floor, such as hardwood
(carpet is too slippery)

Time Needed:
One minute

Instructions:

◎ Start standing tall with the inside edges of your feet touching and your hands on your hips.

◎ Step your feet wide apart and straighten your arms out to your sides at shoulder height—your feet should be directly under your wrists. Bring your hands back to your hips.

◎ Make sure the outer edges of your feet are parallel to each other with all ten toes pointing straight ahead.

◎ Reach down through your feet to ground your energy as you lift the back of your neck up to lengthen your spine.

◎ On an exhale, bend forward at your hips to lower your back parallel to the floor.

◎ Inhale, lengthen your spine here, reaching the crown of your head away from your buttocks and your buttocks away from the crown of your head.

◎ Keeping your hands on your hips and your spine long, exhale and fold your torso down over your legs as far as it will go.

◎ Bring your fingertips to the floor directly underneath your shoulders. Let your head dangle.

◎ Stay here and breathe. On each inhale, lengthen the spine. On each exhale, allow your torso to release farther forward over your legs.

◎ Remain in this pose for ten full breaths.

◎ To come up, softly bend your knees, scoot your feet in toward each other, and slowly roll up to standing, one vertebrae at a time. Bring your head up last.

◎ Go admire that dreamy look in your newly relaxed eyes and the rosy flush on your cheeks.

Modifications:

◎ If your hands don't easily reach the floor, rest them on a stack of books or magazines.

Benefits:

◎ Gives the entire back of your body—legs, buttocks, spine— a nice stretch, which helps relieve tension and makes you better able to enjoy yourself despite your hostess duties

◎ Strengthens the fronts of the legs—all the better to run and fetch some more hors d'oeuvres

◎ Encourages the mind to quiet down so that you can focus on your guests and enjoy yourself instead of thinking of all the other preparations you could have done if you'd had more time

◎ Gently massages and tones your abdominal organs, helping you feel your best

> **Other Remedies to Try:**
> Do-It-Yourself Face Massage
> One-Minute Visualization

Bad Hair Day

No matter what you do, you just don't feel you look your best. Aside from slapping on a headband, is there any way to boost your attractiveness and confidence factor? But of course. . . .

Be warned: This isn't your average beauty advice. It requires you to get down on the floor and do a little bit of playing. The idea is to get you to that place where you radiate because you've been having so much fun and you're feeling comfortable in your own skin. That's when you have a natural beauty that no hairstyle can improve upon. The E! fashion police might not agree, but when is the last time they had any fun? They've been too busy sitting in the hairstylist's chair or getting their eyebrows waxed. ✿

Remedy:
L-Shaped Handstand

Ingredients:
A couple of clear feet of floor space in front of a wall

Time Needed:
Two minutes

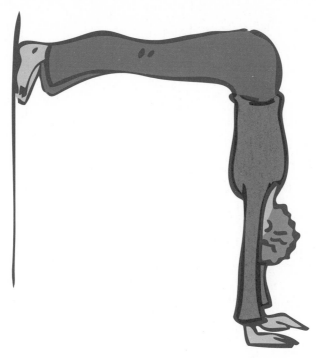

Instructions:

◎ Start on your hands and knees with the soles of your feet touching a wall and your wrists directly underneath your shoulders.

◎ Extend your fingers and bring the entire palm of each hand to the floor.

◎ Straighten your legs to come up into a short upside-down V shape. Your heels can rest an inch or two up the wall.

◎ Reach one foot up the wall to hip height.

◎ Press strongly into that foot and bring your other foot up to meet it, then straighten your legs. Most of your body weight will be on your arms and hands and your body will be in an upside-down L shape.

◎ Reach equally into your hands and feet.

◎ Let your head drop to look at the wall underneath your feet.

◎ Stay here as long as you can—aim for at least five breaths.

◎ To come down, step one foot down to the floor, then the other, and come back to the all-fours position.

◎ Bring your hips to your heels and rest with your forehead on the floor and arms by your sides for a few breaths.

◎ If you're up to it, try it one more time.

Modifications:

◎ If you try the pose and the thought of being upside down is too scary, take the intensity down a notch. Once you've come into the upside-down V shape, lift one leg to rest on the wall as high up as you can reach. Stay there for two or three breaths, then bring that foot down and switch to the other leg. You can try the arm balance another day.

Benefits:

◎ Tones your arms, legs, and torso and makes you feel strong, which is empowering and undeniably sexy

◎ Opens your shoulders, unlocking tension

◎ Imparts the rosy glow that only comes from the perfect combination of exertion and enjoyment

◎ Helps you see things from a new perspective

◎ May even help your hair fall into a more attractive shape

Other Remedies to Try:
Standing Wide-Legged Forward Bend

Public Humiliation

*T*hings were going so well until you went to the bathroom and realized that you have a piece of your lunch wedged firmly between your two front teeth. (Or your fly is down, or you have toilet paper on your shoe, or a glob of spaghetti sauce on your shirt.) You feel embarrassed, maybe a little miffed that no one has told you, and worst of all, you have to go back out there and be your charming self when all you feel like doing is crawling into the nearest hole. Stay strong! First off, remember that no one escapes these little embarrassments. Try to imagine how funny it will be when you recount what happened to your friend, family member, or significant other when you get home. And take sixty seconds to do a simple stretch that opens your heart so that you can avoid total shutdown. Because, let's face it, you're still pretty cute. Even with broccoli in your teeth.

Remedy:
Heart-Opening Stretch

Ingredients:
Two hands

Time Needed:
One minute

Instructions:

🌀 Sit up tall on the edge of your chair (or on the toilet) with both feet flat on the floor, or stand with the back of your neck lifted up.

🌀 Reach your arms behind you and clasp your hands together.

🌀 Straighten your arms so your combined fist is pointing down toward the floor.

🌀 Inhale a deep breath and begin to raise your arms up as you keep your shoulder blades moving down your back.

🌀 With each exhale, imagine blowing any stress you might be feeling out of your body. With each inhale, gently lift your chest and hands a little higher.

🌀 Remain in this pose for ten full breaths.

Modifications:

🌀 If you're in a public place and self-conscious about stretching, you can do this in a bathroom stall.

🌀 If you have difficulty keeping your hands intertwined, hold one end of a scarf or belt in each hand. This will grant you a little more room to maneuver while still giving the front of your torso a nice stretch.

Benefits:

🌀 Opens the heart, which helps you be gentle with yourself, reminds you that you are still completely lovable, and keeps you from shutting down

🌀 Deepens your breathing, which promotes relaxation

Other Remedies to Try:
4-7-8 Breath

Bad Service

A store clerk is rude, or a taxi driver takes you the long way, or a waiter bungles your order and then gets snooty when you point out that you've been waiting an hour for your meal. These undeniably frustrating situations can really stick in your craw because they shine a light on the unpleasant fact that you are not in total control of your life. When you get in a taxi, you can tell the driver where you want to go, but he's the one behind the wheel. Interacting with others requires a small surrender, and when things go awry, you can end up feeling like a sucker.

Just remember that while you may not be able to control people or events, you *can* control the way you react to them. Many people respond to unpleasant interactions by getting huffy and raising their voices. While it's a fairly human reaction to respond to aggression with aggression, this tactic only results in esca-

> While you may not be able to control people or events, you can control the way you react to them.

lating the situation. (It's also awkward at best and embarrassing at worst.) A much better way to respond to the situation is to speak up for yourself while also letting go of any frustration. Remaining calm snuffs out any sparks that might burst into an all-out flame of confrontation. It also models the behavior you'd like to receive and makes you much more likely to get it than screaming or cursing. This breathing exercise is completely unobtrusive, yet it helps you keep your wits about you as you physically release anger and frustration. It's based on a favorite technique of Dr. Andrew Weil and Dr. Tracey Gaudet—I learned it from reading their books, and it has become one of my go-to tools for coping with stressful situations as they arise. 🌸

Remedy:
4-7-8 Breath

Ingredients:
Attention

Time Needed:
As little as ten seconds, or as long as it takes for you to feel less agitated

Instructions:

🌀 Inhale through your nose for a count of four.

🌀 Hold your breath in for a count of seven.

🌀 Exhale through your mouth for a count of eight.

🌀 Repeat as necessary.

Modifications:

🌀 If another count is more comfortable to you, use that instead. Just be sure that you exhale for twice as long as you inhale.

Benefits:

In times of tension, the diaphragm often locks up, resulting in shallow breathing that creates more stress in the body. This cooling breath engages the diaphragm and forces it to work, freeing it from becoming frozen.

Deeper exhales naturally encourage deeper inhales, and deep breathing fosters relaxation.

Exhales always carry things out of the body that you don't need (while inhales are more about infusing the body with new oxygen and energy). Extending the exhalation releases even more undesirable contents, from carbon dioxide to negative emotions.

Counting the length of your breaths promotes focus and keeps your thoughts from spiraling out of control.

Other Remedies to Try:
Lion Pose in the Bathroom
Mini Loving Kindness Meditation

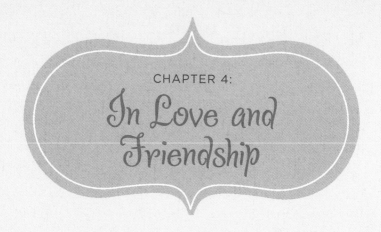

CHAPTER 4:

In Love and Friendship

You might think it would be easiest to stay calm and grounded around the people to whom you are closest. The irony is that the people who know you best are also the most likely to push your buttons. They can't help it—they know you so well and you spend so much time together that you're bound to accidentally bump into each other's sore spots. Think of your loved ones as your own personal gurus, generously and consistently giving you opportunities to practice your dedication to choosing serenity over stress.

Of course, it's not all bad. Your friends and loved ones can also make you laugh like no one else, and they know just how to comfort you when you need a boost. But since this book is about reducing stress, we're going to focus on the sticky situations that will inevitably arise in your personal life. May the following remedies help you smooth any rough edges off your most important relationships and help you become an even better friend, lover, and family member.

Giving Bad News

The task has fallen to you to deliver a piece of bad news, whether it's firing a coworker, telling your girlfriend that you suspect her boyfriend is cheating, or breaking the news to your parents that you won't be home for the holidays. Your first urge may be to cut short that awkward period of anticipation and get the whole business behind you. But there's no sense in making this any worse for the recipient. If you don't have your thoughts gathered, you could ramble on and extend his or her agony. Or, if you're too blunt, you could make the blow sting more than it needs to. Your state of mind will affect how the other person feels as he or she hears the news—if you're shaken, his or her anxiety levels will start rising even before you begin talking. You need to be calm, compassionate, and clear.

> *Your state of mind will affect how the other person feels as he or she hears the news.*

This exercise requires you to breathe as slowly as possible for two full minutes. Coaxing yourself into a slower speed helps you relax and gather your thoughts so that you can deliver the news with a silver spoon instead of a sledgehammer. Do it when you're alone, preferably right before your conversation. ❧

Remedy:
Slow Breath

Ingredients:
A watch or timer (optional)

Time Needed:
Two minutes

Instructions:

◎ Sit up tall in a chair or cross-legged on the floor—a tall spine expands your entire torso, resulting in more room for your lungs to maneuver.

◎ Breathing through your nose, inhale to a count of four and exhale to a count of four.

◎ Gradually extend the length of your inhales and exhales to a count of seven or eight.

◎ When the timer goes off, resume breathing normally.

Modifications:

◎ Using a timer is preferable, because it gives you one less thing to think about. If you're using a timer, set it to two minutes. If you're not, aim to continue the exercise for sixteen full breaths.

◎ Take care not to hold your breath—you want to slow it down, not stop it altogether.

Benefits:

◎ Calms the nervous system, making you better able to deliver the news as serenely as possible

◎ Quiets your thoughts and promotes your focus so that you'll be able to speak clearly and remember everything you want to say

◎ Promotes a noticeable sense of relaxation, which will also put your recipient at ease

> **Other Remedies to Try:**
> Get Grounded • Loving Kindness Meditation

Receiving Bad News

No one wants to anticipate bad news. But stick this tip in your memory bank so that the next time someone asks, "Are you sitting down?," you'll have a technique for keeping it together as you hear that your grandmother needs heart surgery, your roommate is moving out by the end of the month, or that your pet project at work has been shelved.

This easy exercise establishes your connection to the ground, which promotes feelings of stability. That may sound overly simple, but yoga, traditional Chinese medicine, martial arts, and Native American traditions all consider the earth to be a source of personal energy and power. After all, if it weren't for the ground, we'd be eternally adrift at sea or floating through space—not very safe places to be. ❧

Remedy:
Get Grounded

Ingredients:
Your two feet
A chair

Time Needed:
As long as necessary

Instructions:

◎ Sit up tall in your chair.

◎ Uncross your legs and bring the soles of both feet flat on the floor.

◎ Press down gently and evenly across the soles of your feet. You don't need to strain—if your thighs tense up, you've gone too far. Your goal is simply to bring awareness to your connection with the ground.

◎ When you notice that your attention has shifted, which it will, resume consciously checking in on the sensation of your feet planted firmly on the ground.

◎ Repeat as necessary.

Modifications:

◎ You can also do this exercise while standing. Your feet will already be on the floor, obviously, but focus on feeling your weight evenly distributed across the soles of both feet—no cocking your hips and standing with one leg bent.

◎ You can try this anytime you need to stay alert and pay attention—during a business meeting, a phone call, even in the movie theater if you feel yourself getting sleepy.

Benefits:

◎ Shifts your awareness away from your swirling thoughts and into your body, meaning you'll be able to take in information without immediately flying off to Anxiety Land

◎ Gives you something to do that you can control at a time when it may feel that your life is spiraling out of control

Foot-in-Mouth Syndrome

One minute you're gabbing along, the next you realize you've said something that offends your friend. Oops. You've got to gather your wits before you make matters worse.

You don't have a lot of time to react, but don't panic. You just need to give yourself one quiet moment to compose yourself in order to find the right way to apologize or redirect. This simple exercise gives you that moment. It also signals your body to stop pumping out the stress hormones that would otherwise make you likely to react hastily and say something else inappropriate. Best of all, you can do it wherever you are, no matter how many people are around you, in about ten seconds.

> *Give yourself one quiet moment to compose yourself in order to find the right way to apologize or redirect.*

Remedy:
Complete Breath

Ingredients:
A tall spine

Time Needed:
Ten seconds

Instructions:

◎ Be sure that wherever you are, sitting or standing, your spine is lifted up tall so that there's plenty of space in your abdomen and chest for your lungs to expand.

◎ Begin by inhaling into the lower part of your stomach, beneath your belly button.

◎ Continue filling your chest from the low belly to the very tops of your lungs beneath your collarbones. Imagine your torso filling up with air the same way a glass fills up with water—from bottom to top.

◎ Once you've inhaled as much as you can, slowly let the air seep out in reverse order—from the top of your chest, the middle of your rib cage, the area behind your belly button, and your lowest abdomen.

◎ Resume breathing normally.

Modifications:

◎ If you can, place your hand on your belly and feel it move out as you inhale.

◎ Taking even one complete breath can help you find the mental clarity you need to handle the situation, but taking more will only increase the benefit. Take several complete breaths if you need or are able to. Or periodically take a complete breath during the rest of your conversation to ensure that you don't veer back into awkward territory.

Benefits:

◉ Deep breaths unlock the diaphragm, the parachute-shaped muscle that aids in breathing and tends to tighten up during stressful moments. When the diaphragm is tense, it signals the body that all is not well. Releasing it with a conscious exhale is the equivalent of giving the all-clear sign.

◉ This quick remedy gives your brain a micro-vacation—hopefully, just enough time to gather your thoughts.

> **Other Remedies to Try:**
> 4-7-8 Breath • Get Grounded

Asking for Help

Let's face it—women are natural born multitaskers. You may be so busy taking care of everything or so accustomed to handling it all on your own that it doesn't even occur to you to ask for backup. Perhaps you think no one else could get things done to quite the same level that you can, or that it's simply too much bother to explain what you need. Or maybe your reasons run a little deeper—you're afraid that asking for help is a sign of weakness or incompetence, or an admission of defeat. Regardless of your reasoning, it's time to stop the madness! No one gets by without a little help now and then. (Or, sometimes, a truckload of help.)

Not asking for assistance not only makes you less likely to receive the support you need, but it also denies those close to you a chance to show how much they care. It's time for some of those walls to come crumbling down, whether the help you need is a small favor or a substantial request.

This exercise opens your heart and encourages it to lead the way. It's named after the cobra, which has the ability to shed what doesn't serve it anymore and evolve into a better version of itself. Get ready to break out of your stoic habits and leave them in the dust. 🌸

Remedy:
Cobra Pose

Ingredients:
Nonrestrictive and non-lumpy clothes (so you can lie
on your stomach comfortably)
Carpet, towel, or yoga mat to provide padding

Time Needed:
Three minutes

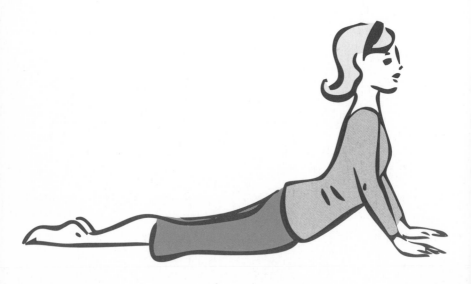

Instructions:

◉ Lie on your stomach on a soft piece of carpet, a towel, or a yoga mat, with the tops of your feet resting on the floor.

◉ Prop yourself up on your forearms with your elbows directly underneath your shoulders.

◉ Look straight ahead.

◉ Press the tops of your feet into the floor to energize your legs.

◉ Imagine reaching your tail bone—the pointy tip of your spine that lies inside the top of your butt crack—down toward your feet to lengthen your lower back. Even if you can't feel anything happening physically, imagining the movement will eventually help your body figure out how to make it happen.

◉ Press into your palms and begin to straighten your arms. As your torso rises, your spine will naturally arch. To ensure that you don't over-arch and cause pain in your lower back, let your chest move forward, away from your feet, as much as you can.

◉ Allow your shoulder blades to slide down your back—the tops of your shoulders will move away from your ears. You will be in a position that's similar to Upward Dog, except your thighs, knees, and calves are resting on the floor.

◉ Once your arms are straight, remain in this position for eight to ten breaths.

◉ Continue looking straight ahead, reaching your chest forward and your tailbone backward, and pressing into the tops of your feet. You want your entire body to be energized, but not tense.

◎ Slowly bend your arms to lower your torso and forehead to the floor.

◎ Turn your cheek to one side and rest for a few breaths; then repeat if you like.

Modifications:

◎ If your lower back feels good in the pose and you'd like to go farther, move your elbows back along the floor, closer to your waist, before you straighten your arms.

◎ If the pose hurts your lower back, move your elbows farther forward, away from your face, to reduce the curve in your lower back during the pose. Focus on reaching your tailbone toward your feet and really extending your chest forward.

◎ Be careful not to over-squeeze your buttocks. Those glute muscles are like the coworker who insists on working on every project—they are busybodies. Their help isn't needed here. In fact, if they're clenched, they'll just tighten your lower back. So let those puppies relax.

Benefits:

◎ Most important, it opens your heart, lungs, upper chest, and throat. This is the area of your body that helps you open up to and communicate with other people.

◎ It simultaneously strengthens and releases tension from the back muscles, making you better able to support yourself so that you don't have to rely on others to do *all* your heavy lifting for you.

🌀 The Cobra Pose stimulates and tones your abdominal organs, which are responsible for, among other things, carrying whatever you don't need out of your body, which in this case could include a resistance to asking for help, embarrassment, or shame.

Other Remedies to Try:
Supported Child's Pose

Saying "No"

Raise your hand if you've ever agreed to something that every bone in your body was telling you to turn down. You are so not alone. (Does anyone still have both hands on this book?) Women in particular are prone to chronically overextending themselves. Saying "no" just seems so . . . impolite. Bitchy, even. The irony is, the more you say yes to things that don't light you up in some way, the less time you have for yourself, and the more frazzled, tired, and cranky you become. And that's when the true bitchiness starts flying.

Imagine your energy is like money. If you give it away to everyone who asks, you won't have any left to buy groceries. A much more efficient way to share your resources—whether it's money, time, or attention—requires that you be choosy. If someone asks you a favor that offers you something in return—satisfaction, enjoyment, an opportunity to learn something new—and you have time and energy to give it your full attention, by all means say yes. But if it will only deplete you by sucking your time, energy, and attention, saying no will actually be doing you and the people around you a favor. The only difficulty is working up the gumption to do it with just the right combination of authority and gentleness.

> *This exercise creates an opportunity for you to hone your strength as well as your vulnerability.*

This exercise creates an opportunity for you to hone your strength as well as your vulnerability. By working your arms and legs while exposing your abdomen, it teaches you that every display of power ("No, I can't rewrite your resume for you . . .") is best accompanied by an equal measure of humility ("but I'm honored you asked and I would be happy to take a look at your first draft."). When you can combine the two, saying "no" allows you to set boundaries for yourself without turning into a total ice queen. 🌸

Remedy:
Goddess Pose

Ingredients:
Bare feet

Time Needed:
Two minutes

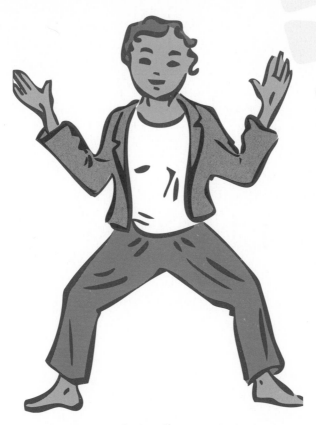

Instructions:

🌀 Stand with your legs about three feet apart, toes turned out slightly.

🌀 Bring your arms straight out to your sides at shoulder height. Bend your elbows so they are a few inches outside your waist and your hands are at shoulder height, palms facing out.

🌀 Bend your knees into a plié.

⊚ Stay here, with knees bent and arms up, and breathe slow, deep breaths through your nose.

⊚ After five breaths, bend your knees a little deeper. You should feel your thighs burning. Keep your hands, chest, and head high—you want to take up as much space all around you as you can. Aim to take five more breaths here, working right up to your physical limit. (Quaking legs are a good sign that you're at your edge—hang in there and continue breathing.)

⊚ After ten total breaths, straighten your legs and lower your arms.

⊚ Rest for a few moments; then repeat the pose one more time.

Modifications:

⊚ If you'd like to increase the intensity, incorporate thirty seconds of quick inhalations and exhalations through the nose (known as the breath of fire) during your pose. It will help turn up the flame on your will to say "no." If you try this, keep your breath light and staccato, like a dog panting.

Benefits:

⊚ Reminds you that you have every right to claim time and space for yourself—something we as women too often forget

⊚ Strengthens your arms and legs, making you better able to walk toward and reach for what you want and need

◎ Gives you a glimpse of the reserves of strength you possess and teaches you to hold your ground

◎ Reminds you that it's possible to be strong and vulnerable at the same time, helping you to say no with grace instead of pure aggression

---

Other Remedies to Try:
Inflate Yourself

Family Gatherings

Invariably, your least favorite uncle will ask prying questions about your love life, your Great-Aunt Jean will clear her throat incessantly at the dinner table, and your mom will make a comment about your hair. Taken together, it might be enough to set your eye to twitching, make you snappy, or get you reaching for one too many glasses of wine or helpings of dessert. While you can't stop the people you love from doing the things that drive you crazy, you *can* change your reaction to them.

It might even help you enjoy the togetherness instead of simply enduring it.

Before your next family gathering, make a mental list of the behaviors that typically trigger your stress reaction. Once you're in the thick of the proceedings, vow to repeat a simple mantra as you take a deep breath each time one of your triggers occurs. Breathing deeply helps your body relax, while the mantra gives your mind something to focus on other than the annoying behavior, lessening its sting. It creates little opportunities for you to release stress before you react out of anger. And it might even help you enjoy the togetherness instead of simply enduring it. 🌸

Remedy:
Mantra Meditation

Ingredients:
A favorite word or phrase

Time Needed:
Intermittent bursts of a few seconds

Instructions:

◎ Before the big event, choose a favorite word or phrase to use as your mantra, such as "pure love," "amen," "bless his (or her) heart," "peace," or even "forgive them, Father." It could be any phrase—the only requirement is that it has meaning to you.

◎ Make a mental list of the behaviors that trip your wires.

◎ When you're at the gathering, every time one of your triggers occurs, take a full inhale and full exhale, repeating your mantra silently as you do. Promise yourself you won't speak, roll your eyes, or otherwise react until you've given yourself a few seconds to repeat your mantra.

Modifications:

🌀 Family gatherings are a particularly great place to practice this technique, because family dynamics can be so darn predictable and so desperately in need of a change. But you can use this technique during any stressful situation—a job interview, a difficult conversation with a loved one, a traffic jam, and so on.

Benefits:

🌀 Taking a moment to de-stress before you respond to a rude comment from your Uncle Larry will likely help defuse the situation rather than escalate it, resulting in a more pleasant evening for everyone involved.

🌀 Repeating a mantra gives your thoughts a moment to rest before springing into action, making you more likely to react calmly.

🌀 A deep breath signals your body that the stress has passed, helping you relax even in the midst of an otherwise tense moment.

Other Remedies to Try:
Chamomile Tea • Complete Breath

Dumping Someone

reakups aren't easy, whether you're the dumper or the dumpee. After all, even though you don't want to continue dating, you do care about this person (at least, you did up until recently) and don't want to hurt his or her feelings. But you also need to be clear and firm that it's time for you both to move on. In order to communicate what needs to be said without being ruthless, you have to strike a delicate balance between gentleness and precision.

This exercise teaches you how to walk that balance with yourself, making you much more likely to be able to achieve it in your interactions with another person. It may seem overly simple—count to five, then start again. But you will get distracted, and you will lose count. It's human nature for the mind to wander. The true lesson of this meditation is to learn how to stay calm and loving when things go awry and to practice simply starting again—two traits that will serve you well during the conversation itself and in the days and weeks that follow. Try it before you work out what you're going to say or just before the final conversation. It will help you make a clean break with compassion. 🌸

Remedy:
Three-Minute Meditation

Ingredients:
Timer or clock

Time Needed:
Three minutes

Instructions:

🌀 Sit comfortably in a chair or on the floor. You want to able to sit still for three full minutes—use pillows to prop yourself up or sit back in your chair to support your spine.

🌀 Set a timer for three minutes so that you can relieve yourself from having to monitor the clock. If you don't have a timer, notice your start time.

🌀 Begin by focusing your attention on the sensation of your breathing for a few breaths. Feel your chest rise and fall, or the air flowing inside your nostrils—whatever detail is easiest for you to notice.

🌀 Once you've settled into a calmer state of mind, begin silently counting each exhale. Start with one and work your way up to five.

🌀 After you've counted your fifth exhale, start again with one on your next breath.

🌀 If you find that you've lost count or reached ten breaths without noticing, simply start again at one. No berating yourself allowed.

🌀 Continue counting five exhales at a time until the timer goes off or you see that three minutes have passed.

🌀 Once your time is up, breathe normally for a few moments before resuming normal life.

Modifications:

🌀 You can keep your eyes open or closed, whichever suits you best. If you're tired and closing your eyes only makes you sleepier, keep them open. If you're amped up and can't keep your eyes from looking around the room, close them.

Benefits:

◎ The structure of this exercise teaches you how to start over when you get off track—a trait that will keep you from rambling as you're delivering the news.

◎ It cultivates focus, which will come in handy as you determine what you want to say.

◎ Counting your exhales fosters a sense of calm so that you can speak clearly and openly.

◎ Finally, it teaches you how to simply move on when things go wrong instead of getting involved in a lot of drama—something you and your former paramour will appreciate immensely now and in the future.

> **Other Remedies to Try:**
> Cobra Pose • Get Grounded

Getting Dumped

Oof. Even if you secretly know it's for the best, it still smarts. You startle yourself awake during your first post-breakup nights because you wandered over to the empty side of the bed. You fear you'll never have sex again. You wonder what you'll do on national holidays.

Although it's not comfortable to be healing from a broken heart, there is something beautiful about being recently broken-up. It's an opportunity to reshape your life—you can now do whatever you want with whomever you please. Isn't there a new bar or restaurant you've been wanting to try but never did because your ex pooh-poohed it? Or a favorite shirt you haven't worn since you first started dating because the two of you spent most nights on the couch watching *Law & Order?* Surely there's *something* you can look forward to.

You're in an awkward position—not ready to crawl under the covers for the next two years, but not ready to move forward yet either. It's natural to want to rush through these times of transition so that you can feel like you again. But the quickest way to end the post-breakup wonkiness is to acknowledge that you're going through a weird time and then embrace that awkward feeling.

> *It may not look pretty, but it's a great way to practice feeling strong and steady.*

Here's an exercise that requires you to get into a challenging and ungainly position—somewhere between sitting and standing—and then hold it. It may not look pretty, but it's a great way to practice feeling strong and steady but still open to whatever the future may bring. It helps you not only accept your transitional state but also own it and feel stronger for it. The Sanskrit translation for this exercise is "fierce pose"—spend a few minutes here and you'll quickly realize that you have stores of power you may not have ever previously tapped. Those same stores will see you through this rough, yet finite, time. Prepare to rock the awkwardness! 🌸

Remedy:
Awkward Pose

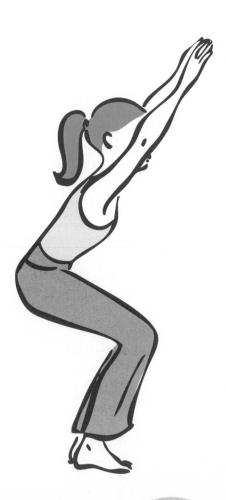

Ingredients:
Wall (optional)

Time Needed:
Three minutes

Instructions:

◎ Stand with your feet hips' distance apart.

◎ Reach your arms up as high as you can, elbows straight, with your hands about twelve inches apart and palms facing each other.

◎ Inhale a deep breath and lift your rib cage up off your waist.

◎ Exhale and drop your shoulder blades down your back.

◎ Bend your knees deeply and let your tush move down and out behind you as if you were about to sit on an invisible chair.

◎ Choose something at eye level to look at. Having something to focus on helps cultivate your determination to "see it through."

◎ Stay here and breathe. Awkward, isn't it? Remember . . . breathe! You're here to learn how to become comfortable in an uncomfortable situation. Holding your breath is not comfortable.

◎ Find a balance between exerting effort and relaxing into the pose: Keep reaching out through your fingertips and the sides of your body while your pelvis and your thighs get heavy and move down toward the floor.

◎ Stay for at least five slow, deep breaths.

◎ To come back to standing, straighten your legs and bring your arms down by your sides.

◎ Repeat three times.

Modifications:

◎ If this pose makes you out-and-out miserable, stand two to three feet away from a wall. When you bend your knees, let your backside rest on the wall.

Benefits:

◎ Opens the shoulders, one of the first places stress and fear accumulate

◎ Strengthens the ankles and legs, giving you a sturdy foundation

◎ Broadens the chest and heart, helping you remain open to new experiences

◎ Helps you feel grounded or rooted, even when it feels like the earth is moving underneath you.

Other Remedies to Try:
Heart Meditation • Self-Massage
Supported Heart Opener • Warrior's Breath

Fight with Husband/Boyfriend/ Family Member/Friend

This is one of the most important people in your life and you've both just said some things to each other that sting. There's no turning back now—the only way your relationship is going to recover is by moving forward. But right now, your chest is heaving, your face is flushed, and your emotions are raging. You have to find a way to dissipate the riled-up energy that's coursing through your body. Sitting and breathing is not going to cut it!

You need to do something with your body that also helps you calm down and concentrate. This exercise helps do just that. Best of all, you can do it wherever you are for as little or as long as you like—whatever it takes for you to start feeling better. And you will start feeling better soon. Don't let this upset convince you otherwise. ❧

Remedy:
Walking Meditation

Ingredients:
Bare feet (preferable, but not required)
A somewhat quiet, obstacle-free place to walk

Time Needed:
As little as one minute, or as many
as fifteen or twenty

Instructions:

- Start standing with the inside edges of your feet touching.

- Turn both your hands palm up and rest your dominant hand in your nondominant hand.

- Bring both hands to rest just below your belly button.

- Cast your gaze on the floor a few feet ahead of you.

- As slowly as you can, peel your right foot off the floor and place it approximately one foot in front of its starting position.

- Feel every sensation as you transfer your weight to your right foot—how your left foot lifts off the floor a little at a time, how your center of gravity shifts forward.

- Continue taking one mindful step at time. Take care to feel the ground beneath your feet (being barefoot helps) and the shifting sensations in your body as you do.

- Notice when you feel the urge to rush, or when something distracts you. Then just continue putting one foot in front of the other.

- Keep walking until you feel calmer, clearer, and more grounded.

Modifications:

- Although it would be ideal to do this outside where the fresh air will further placate your nerves, it's also great to do inside. If you're walking in a hallway and reach a wall, simply turn around and reverse directions. Or walk in a circle around your living room. It's not about getting somewhere—it's about noticing each step.

🌀 This is great to do anytime you have nervous energy to burn and need help calming down. You can even do it on your way to the bathroom, making it a great way to build a little mindfulness into even the most hectic day.

Benefits:

🌀 Helps your mind and body slow down, making you less likely to spiral into a full-blown tizzy

🌀 Physically removes you from a heated situation, giving you the space you need to obtain a little clarity

🌀 Gives you something to do with your body that requires little time and preparation—as opposed to, say, going to the gym—while you quiet your thoughts

🌀 Reminds you not to take the simple things for granted (If you can remember what a miracle it is to be able to walk wherever you like, perhaps you can also remember the little things the person you're fighting with has done for you.)

Other Remedies to Try:
Invisible Trampoline
Lion Pose in the Bathroom • Powerful Breath

Apologizing

When you accidentally bump into someone on the street, or dial a wrong number, or drop your pencil during a meeting, apologizing is effortless, even compulsive. But when the stakes get higher—you betray someone's trust, for example—apologizing becomes a totally different exercise. You can't mindlessly murmur, "I'm sorry," and expect it to carry any weight. You have to take a risk and convey your truest feelings as you ask for forgiveness in order to restore trust with the person you've hurt. It's not always easy, but it is possible.

This exercise can help facilitate the sincere communication that starts to mend any broken bridges. It works by opening your heart, the location of your fourth chakra, and the throat, home of the fifth chakra. Yogis believe the fourth chakra governs our ability to love ourselves and others while the fifth chakra rules our ability to communicate with others, express our emotions, and listen. Sounds like just what the doctor ordered for this situation, no? Get ready to lay down some truth and prove Elton John wrong—sorry doesn't always have to be the hardest word. 🌸

Remedy:
Baby Camel Pose

Ingredients:
Carpet or yoga mat
Nonbinding clothes

Time Needed:
Three minutes

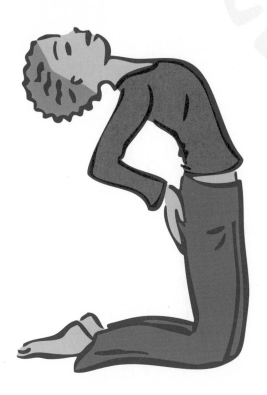

Instructions:

◎ Kneel on the floor with your knees directly under your hips—there should be about a fist's distance between your knees.

◎ Untuck your toes so that the tops of your feet are on the floor.

◎ Bring your hands to the back of your hips—palms resting on the tops of your buttocks and fingers pointing down toward the floor.

◎ Reach your elbows toward each other to open your chest.

◎ Reach down through the tops of your feet and your shins as you lift the crown of your head up to unfurl your entire spine.

◎ Keep lifting so strongly that you begin to arch your upper back backward.

◎ Arch back as far as you can while keeping your thighs and hips reaching forward.

◎ Let your head drop back (if it's comfortable for you) and feel your throat yawn open.

◎ Remain in this position for five to ten breaths.

◎ To come up, press strongly down into your shins as you lead with your chest to come back to the starting position.

◎ Lower your hips to your heels and head to the floor to rest for a moment before resuming normal activity.

Modifications:

◎ If the pose is easy for you and you'd like to turn up the intensity, tuck your toes under and reach for your ankles with your hands (instead of keeping them on your butt). You'll get a bigger opening across the chest and throat. Just remember to keep reaching up strongly through your chest so that you don't cause too much stress on your lower back.

◎ If it's uncomfortable for you to allow your head to fall back, point your chin, face, and gaze straight up at the ceiling. Do reach the crown of your head away from your shoulders so your neck and throat can be nice and long.

Benefits:

◎ Stretches the entire front of the body—ankles, calves, thighs, abdomen, chest, and throat—making you more supple and better able to be the flexible one in your exchange

◎ Strengthens the back, meaning you don't have to compromise your integrity even though you are "bending over backward" to make amends with someone

◎ Teaches you how to lead with your heart and allow your throat to be open so that you can more easily express your truest feelings

◎ Massages and stimulates the kidneys and adrenal glands, helping you regulate your stress levels (The adrenals sit right above the kidneys in your lower back and are the source of the hormones your body produces when it's stressed. Compressing the adrenals during the backbend encourages fresh blood to flow into them, washing away any stale blood and gently toning them.)

Other Remedies to Try:
Cobra Pose • Loving Kindness Meditation
Three-Minute Meditation

Forgiveness

When someone has done you wrong, you may feel tempted to hate that person forever or to avoid him or her for the rest of your natural born days. Either option seems a lot easier than sorting through the thorny emotions that his or her transgression has stirred up. The problem with this logic is that forgiveness is a crucial ingredient for your own well-being. It's nearly impossible to move on and grow without it. Although it can be undeniably difficult to forgive someone who has hurt you, the good news is that it does become easier with practice.

> *Forgiveness is a crucial ingredient for your own well-being.*

The purpose of this exercise isn't to force forgiveness to happen. It's to open the door and invite it to arrive on its own. With a little mental discipline and the power of suggestion, you'll take important steps toward liberation from the ill will that would otherwise fester like an impacted tooth. Let the healing begin! ❧

Remedy:
Forgiveness Meditation

Ingredients:
Quiet
Privacy

Time Needed:
Three to five minutes, as needed

Instructions:

◎ Sit comfortably either in a chair or on the floor. To make sure you don't get distracted by the physical effort of holding yourself upright, use pillows to support yourself if you're sitting on the floor or scoot back so that your whole spine can rest on the back of the chair.

◎ Close your eyes and take a few moments to acquaint yourself with the sensation of your breath.

◎ Once your thoughts have quieted a bit, call up an image of the person who has hurt you.

◎ Really see the details of his or her face to make the experience as real as possible.

◎ As you do this, silently repeat to yourself "I forgive you" as many times as you'd like.

◎ If there's more than one person involved, repeat the above step for each of them.

◎ With each inhale, think of breathing in compassion, acceptance, or warmth—whatever feels right to you. As you exhale, imagine blowing out resentment, anger, or hurt.

◎ Keep going until you feel a shift. Let's face it, you're probably not going to experience total euphoria or complete peace. But perhaps you'll notice that your chest isn't as heavy, or your face as flushed. That's a cue that something has started to lift.

◎ Spend a few quiet moments simply breathing before you open your eyes.

◎ Repeat as often as necessary.

Benefits:

◉ Helps you practice the messy art of forgiveness (While it may not result in a spontaneous release from all anguish, it will help you get better at the process of releasing old hurts.)

◉ Cultivates your compassion, an essential component of forgiveness

◉ Gives you an opportunity to let all of your negative emotions rise to the surface and a means to usher them along

Other Remedies to Try:
Heart Meditation
Loving Kindness Meditation

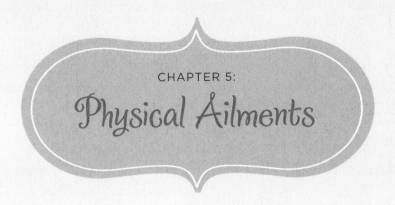

CHAPTER 5:

Physical Ailments

You may not realize it, but your body regularly communicates with you. All day, every day, it sends signals that are designed to inform you of what it needs to function. Hunger pangs are a clear example—when your stomach grumbles, it's time to refuel. But other signs may not be so obvious to you. A sore back can indicate that you're pushing yourself too hard; hiccups that you're emotionally upset; PMS that you're not giving yourself enough downtime.

While none of the remedies in this chapter are a guaranteed, now-and-forever "cure," they all empower you to take control of your own day-to-day physical well-being by providing a means for engaging in a dialogue with yourself. With them, when your body presents a symptom, you no longer have to resign yourself to suffer through it or take a pill and hope for the best. You can try the technique suggested here, which sends a message to your body that says, "I hear you, and I'm here to help." Once your body knows that you're listening, it won't have to talk quite so loudly to get your attention, and you'll become better able to recognize the signals your body sends and respond to them before things get out of hand. As an added bonus, since your body and mind are inextricably linked, when you take better care of your physical health, your mental health will follow.

Hangover

What doesn't feel funky? Your stomach is churning, your head is aching, your hands are shaking. Your energy level is at an all-time low, and about the only activity that sounds remotely appealing is watching bad daytime television while eating a bucket of fries. Not that there's anything wrong with that course of action. But you can try a few more proactive remedies to usher that sick feeling along, which will likely result in your feeling better, sooner.

First, drink water. Alcohol dehydrates your body, which only exacerbates your physical woes and mental fog. Drinking water alleviates symptoms associated with dehydration as it also helps the body flush excess alcohol and alcohol by-products from the system. Get yourself a pitcher of cool water and a glass and start sipping, refilling as necessary.

Once you've covered this basic step, move on to the remedy—a delicious banana milk shake that will replenish the stores of fructose, potassium, magnesium, and B vitamins that your alcohol intake has decimated. (It can't hurt to stock up on bananas before a night out on the town . . . just in case.) Then, when you feel you've bolstered your strength, take as brisk a walk as you can manage. The fresh air will invigorate you and the exercise will boost your circulation and encourage further release of toxins. *Then* you can doze off on the couch while Judge Judy explains the basic rules of decorum to another hapless oaf. ❀

Remedy:
Banana Milk Shake

Ingredients:
One or two bananas
Milk or soy milk
Honey
Ice cubes (optional)

Time Needed:
Five minutes

Instructions:
🌀 Peel the banana (or two—your choice) and place it (them) in the blender.

🌀 Pour in milk or soy milk to cover the banana(s).

🌀 Squeeze in a tablespoon or so of honey to taste.

🌀 If a cold shake sounds more refreshing, drop in a handful of ice cubes—but be warned, it will make the blending process a whole lot louder.

🌀 Pour the shake into a glass, retreat to the sofa, and enjoy.

Modifications:
🌀 If the sound of the blender is too much for your tender ears to bear, slice the banana, spread it on a piece of whole-grain toast, and drizzle with honey. If that's too much effort, just eat the banana. (And drink your water!)

Benefits:

◎ Bananas and honey are both good sources of the natural sugar fructose, which helps your body process any alcohol remaining in your system and increases your energy level.

◎ Bananas contain magnesium, potassium, and B vitamins—the very nutrients that a night of overimbibing depletes.

◎ Bananas will also soothe your roiling stomach.

> **Other Remedies to Try:**
> Hot Ginger Tea • Stimulate the Union Valley

Headache

Whether it's a dull throb or more of a pounding, headaches are most often caused by tight muscles in the neck, shoulders, and jaw, and are frequently exacerbated by stress. Chinese medicine also believes that headaches are triggered by an excess amount of energy and blood flow in the head. It may be tempting to reach for an over-the-counter pain reliever, but you'll be missing an opportunity to address the root cause of your headache and eliminate it once and for all.

This acupressure exercise targets a point that is associated with the face, neck, jaw, and head. Stimulating this point works to relieve muscular tension that might be contributing to your headache. And because the point is located in your hand, it also helps draw excess energy down from your head and into your extremities, eliminating another root of the pain. You can do it anywhere you can sit or lie quietly. Try it before you head for the medicine cabinet—it will likely save you a trip. As you do the exercise, notice if your thoughts turn to a particular worry. It may well be one of the reasons you got a headache in the first place. When you're feeling better, take some action to rectify the situation.

Important note: Don't stimulate this point if you are pregnant, as practitioners of Chinese Medicine believe it could lead to premature uterine contractions. Try the other remedies listed below instead. ❋

Remedy:
Stimulate the Union Valley

Ingredients:
Thumb and index finger

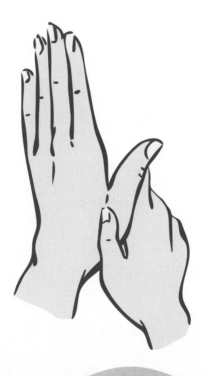

Time Needed:

Two to three minutes

Instructions:

⌾ Locate your Union Valley by extending all the fingers of your left hand and bringing your left thumb right in alongside your left index finger. Union Valley is located in the small mound of flesh just below the bottom of the crease formed by the inner edge of your thumb

⌾ Place your right thumb on your left Union Valley and your right index finger on your left palm directly underneath your right thumb, then let the left hand relax.

⌾ Gently squeeze your right thumb and index finger toward each other to apply moderate pressure to Union Valley on your left hand. Stay here for twenty to thirty seconds, breathing deeply as you do.

⌾ Repeat on the right hand.

Modifications:

⌾ Be careful not to squeeze too hard. You want to tenderly nudge your body toward feeling better, not beat it into submission.

Benefits:

⌾ Applying pressure to any point in the body encourages new blood to flow into the area once the pressure is released. This influx brings in more oxygen and nutrients as it sweeps away stagnant waste products.

◉ As opposed to taking an aspirin or other pain medication, this exercise treats the muscle tightness that is the likely cause of the headache, not just the symptoms.

◉ Breathing deeply as you apply pressure also triggers the body's relaxation response, helping to alleviate the stress that may be a source of the headache in the first place.

◉ This remedy teaches you how to start heeding your body's clues that it needs a little TLC.

Other Remedies to Try:
Head Down Time Out
Supported Seated Forward Bend
Tennis Ball Massage

Upset Stomach

Your stomach is gurgling like Mt. Saint Helen's on the verge of an eruption. It's possible it's the sushi you ate for lunch. Or your jeans are too tight. Or stress is calling your name again. Regardless of the cause, you have an ally in a little herb called ginger. This brown, knobby root won't win any beauty contests, but it packs a wallop of healthful benefits, particularly for anything related to digestion.

Herbalists have used ginger for centuries to treat nausea, seasickness, and cramps. Best of all, it's not

This brown, knobby root won't win any beauty contests, but it packs a wallop of healthful benefits.

some chalky pink concoction that you have to choke down—it makes a tasty cup of tea that gets even more delicious with a squeeze of honey and lemon. Next time you're at the grocery store, pick up two boxes of ginger tea—one for home, one for the office—and brew yourself a cup whenever you're experiencing stomach funkiness. While no herbal remedy can completely replace the care of a trained health provider, taking the time to prepare a remedy for yourself makes you an active participant in your own well-being—and the good feeling that provides can help alleviate some of the stress that may have triggered your stomach upset in the first place.

Note: Although you might be tempted to quell your queasiness with ginger ale, gingersnaps, or gingerbread, these treats—while delicious—are more sugar than healing herb. ❀

Remedy:
Hot Ginger Tea

Ingredients:
Packaged ginger tea bags
Hot water
Honey
A slice of fresh lemon

Time Needed:
Five minutes

Instructions:
◎ Unwrap a tea bag, two if you're really feeling awful, and place it in an empty mug.

◎ Boil water.

◎ Pour the water into the mug and let the tea steep three to four minutes.

◎ Sweeten with honey to taste and add a squeeze of fresh lemon. These additions not only taste great but also boost the tea's effectiveness: Honey has natural antibacterial properties, and lemon's astringency stimulates the production of saliva, which kick-starts the digestive process.

◎ Enjoy, and repeat as necessary.

Modifications:

◎ Ginger can be an acquired taste. If you don't find it deliciously spicy, add more honey and lemon.

◎ Ginger is considered a warming herb, meaning it can be stimulating. If you're already pretty fiery—you get night sweats, have insomnia, acid reflux, ulcers, or chronic acid indigestion—don't drink ginger tea before going to bed. It can still relieve your upset stomach; you should just drink it earlier in the day.

Benefits:

◎ Ginger reduces nausea, vomiting, motion sicknesses, and seasickness. To sweeten the deal, it also relieves flatulence.

◎ It is also believed to help break up and reduce phlegm as well as sore throat pain—try a steaming cup of ginger tea the next time you have a cold.

◎ Ginger can reduce inflammation and thin the blood— good news for sufferers of inflammatory conditions such as rheumatoid arthritis and heart disease.

> **Other Remedies to Try:**
> Banana Milk Shake
> Center of Power Stimulation
> Chamomile Tea • Rock Pose

Constipation

It doesn't matter how brightly the sun may be shining outside. If your digestion isn't working, it feels like there's a permanent little black cloud over your head. Bowels are a sensitive and complex ecosystem. They can get thrown off by stress, illness, travel, even a small change in daily routine. Although there is some mystery as to how digestion works or why it suddenly decides to go on strike, there are a few basic self-care techniques that can help everyone keep things moving.

When your bowels slow to a crawl, prioritize drinking more water, a crucial component that helps usher food through the digestive tract, and getting more exercise. You don't have to kill yourself at the gym, but make sure you are up and moving around for at least thirty minutes a day to stimulate your metabolism. The final ingredient for getting back on track is good old-fashioned fiber. That doesn't mean you have to resort to eating cereal that looks and tastes like twigs. Instead, you can sprinkle flaxseeds, a fabulous source of fiber, on any food. Not just an emergency measure, they can be a part of your daily diet to help you get regular and stay that way.

Note: In order for your body to be able to digest the seeds and reap their benefits, they must be ground up into a fine powder, not eaten whole. See the instructions below for how to grind them. ✿

Remedy:
Ground Flaxseeds

Ingredients:
Flaxseeds, either whole or ground (available in most grocery stores and health food stores near the whole-wheat flour and other grains)

Time Needed:
Seconds to sprinkle over food, slightly longer if you need to grind them first

Instructions:

◎ If your flaxseeds are whole, use a mini-chopper or coffee grinder (preferably an extra one that you don't use to grind coffee, because coffee's strong oils will taint the taste) to pulse them into a powder.

◎ Sprinkle one to two tablespoons over yogurt, salads, cereal, or pasta, or in a smoothie once a day.

◎ Because of the seeds' high fiber content, drink plenty of water when you take them to keep them moving through your digestive tract.

Modifications:

🌀 The seeds have a mild, slightly nutty taste that you probably won't notice. If you don't like the texture, which can be gritty, mix the seeds into something thicker, such as yogurt or chili.

🌀 Store seeds—ground or whole—in the refrigerator or freezer to keep the oil in the seeds from going rancid.

Benefits:

🌀 Two tablespoons of flaxseeds contain just over five grams of fiber—that's 20 percent of your recommended daily intake in one fell swoop.

🌀 They are also an excellent source of omega-3 fatty acids, which have been linked to reducing depression, risk of heart disease, PMS, and allergies while improving memory, eyesight, and brain function.

Other Remedies to Try:
Probiotics • Seated Spinal Twist
Sphinx Pose

Food Coma

Your last meal was so delicious, or you were so ravenous, or so in need of distraction, that you've gone and eaten way too much food. Now your belly feels uncomfortably full and you're overcome with an attack of sluggishness. Whoops. Unbutton your pants and spend a few minutes sitting in this super-simple pose. Yogis refer to it as "rock pose" because they believe you could even digest a rock while seated this way. Coupled with some deep breathing, it's a great way to facilitate digestion. ✿

Remedy:
Rock Pose

Ingredients:
Blanket and/or towel, as needed for comfort

Time Needed:
Five minutes

Instructions:
◎ Kneel with your shins on the floor, toes untucked.

◎ Lower your seat to rest on your heels. Your heels can splay out slightly.

◎ Bring your hands to your belly.

◎ Sit here and feel your belly rise and hands move away from your spine as you inhale and your stomach deflate and hands fall back toward your spine as you exhale.

◎ Remain in this pose at least one full minute, and up to five minutes.

◎ Don't immediately pop back up to standing—your feet may have fallen asleep while you were sitting. Shift your hips to one side and straighten your legs out in front of you for a moment before standing up.

Modifications:

◎ If this is painful on your feet or ankles, fold up a blanket, place it on the floor, and position your shins on the blanket so that your feet hang off the back edge. This will decrease the stretch and pressure on the tops of your feet.

◎ If it hurts your knees, roll up a washcloth or hand towel into a tight little bundle and place it directly behind your knees before you sit back. It will create more space in the knee joint.

◎ Try both of the above modifications if the pose is generally uncomfortable, but do stick with it even if it's only for a breath or two at a time. The more often you sit this way, the more flexible your feet, ankles, and knees will become and the less discomfort you will feel.

Benefits:

◎ The deep breathing gently massages your abdominal organs and helps move things along the digestive tract.

◎ This exercise builds a little active rest into your day, allowing your body to focus on digestion.

> **Other Remedies to Try:**
> Chamomile Tea • Hot Ginger Tea
> Seated Spinal Twist

Hiccups

Hiccups are caused by spasms in your diaphragm—the mushroom-shaped muscle that drapes across the bottom of your rib cage—and boy, do they make you feel spastic when they strike. With their accompanying loud noises and full-body tremors, an attack of the hiccups can make you want to crawl under the nearest table. This mortification doesn't do one thing to alleviate the hiccups, which often come when you're already stressed or upset and breathing erratically due to your mental state—as if the needle on your breathing record gets bumped out of its groove and starts skipping.

When you're in this state, the last thing you need is someone trying to "scare" the hiccups out of you. (Talk about stressful!) Getting scared, drinking water, holding your breath, and most of the other various folk remedies for hiccups are all different ways of changing your breathing patterns and coaxing your diaphragm out of its rhythmic rut. There is a kinder, gentler way. With a combination of deep breathing and a little well-placed acupressure, you'll be on your way to breathing normally in no

> *When you're in this state, the last thing you need is someone trying to "scare" the hiccups out of you.*

time. The acupressure point most associated with hiccups is known as your Windscreen, and it's located directly behind your earlobe. ✿

Remedy:
Apply Pressure to Your Windscreen

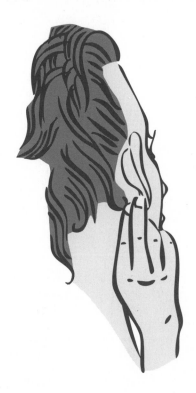

Ingredients:
Your index and middle fingers

Time Needed:
One minute

Instructions:

◎ Find the soft spot right behind each earlobe.

◎ Press your index and middle fingers steadily into this area on both sides of your head—it may be tender, so be gentle yet firm.

◎ Breathe deeply for one minute, allowing your belly to inflate on the inhale and flatten on the exhale.

◎ Gradually release the pressure.

Modifications:

◎ Because hiccups are spasms of the diaphragm, continue breathing deeply after you complete the exercise to keep the diaphragm expanding and contracting rhythmically and nudge it out of its spastic tendencies.

◎ Holding this point also relieves jaw and ear pain and sore throats.

Benefits:

◎ Encourages relaxation, which alleviates the muscle spasms responsible for hiccups

◎ Promotes deep breathing, which encourages the diaphragm to move in a more fluid, less herky-jerky, way

◎ Gives you a sense of control in a situation where it can feel like your body has a mind of its own

> **Other Remedies to Try:**
> Belly Breathing

Insomnia

r. Sandman has lost your number and he's left you crying for a little shut-eye. Insomnia takes different forms—either you can't fall asleep to begin with, or you can fall asleep fine but you wake up in the middle of the night. This remedy can help with either type.

This simple breathing technique is particularly well-suited for helping you get back to sleep for three reasons: First of all, you can do it even when you're lying in bed and exhausted, which is incredibly convenient. Second, taking a longer exhale requires a little act of surrender and helps you purge any tension you may be feeling. And finally, counting the length of your inhale and exhale is just enough of a distraction to take your attention off your thoughts. ✿

> *Taking a longer exhale . . . helps you purge any tension you may be feeling.*

Remedy:
Extended Exhale Breathing

Ingredients:
Two pillows—one for under your head, one for under your knees

Time Needed:
As much time as you like

Instructions:

◎ Lie on your back. Place one pillow under your knees so that you feel extra comfortable and supported. This arrangement also encourages the muscles in your lower back and abdomen to release completely, which enables you to breathe more deeply. The other pillow goes under your head.

◎ Rest your hands on your belly and spend a few breaths feeling your hands rise as you inhale and fall on the exhale.

◎ Once this belly breathing has helped you calm down a little, begin counting the length of your inhales and exhales.

◎ Inhale for a count of four, and exhale for a count of eight.

◎ If this count causes you any stress or strain, modify it to a more appropriate length for you. The only parameter is that the exhale should be twice as long as the inhale.

◎ Repeat until you feel yourself getting sleepy, verrrrry sleeeeeepyyyy. . . .

Modifications:

◎ If you've been at it for twenty minutes and you're still not sleeping, get out of bed. On those long, dark nights when your mind won't quiet down, get up, go in the other room, and write in your journal. It may not make any sense when you look at it by the light of day, but sitting and releasing all the thoughts that are swirling around eventually allows your natural urge for sleep to have its voice heard.

Benefits:

◉ Soothes your nerves, which paves the way for the unrestricted breathing and total muscle relaxation that sleep brings

◉ Gives you something to focus on besides your anxious thoughts and quiets your mind, making you more receptive to sleep's gentle whispers

> **Other Remedies to Try:**
> Chamomile Tea • Open Your Inner Gate
> Rescue Remedy • Supported Child's Pose

No Sleep

Sleep wouldn't come despite your efforts and you spent most of the night awake. Everyone has those endless nights from time to time, when you feel you're the only person on Earth who's awake and your thoughts won't stop swirling. The good news? Your restless night is over. The bad news? You have a full day ahead of you and your energy level is hovering somewhere around the elevation of Death Valley.

Your morning shower can take you a long way toward feeling awake and ready for anything. But not if you luxuriate under a stream of warm, steamy water—a hot shower, no matter how good it may sound, will only leave you dehydrated, noodly, and ready to crawl back under the covers. Instead, take your normal shower and finish by alternating between the coldest water you can stand and lukewarm water. It might be shocking at first, but the energy boost will last for hours. Plus, it's (mostly) free. ❀

Remedy:
Hot/Cold Water Therapy

Ingredients:
Shower

Time Needed:
An additional two to three minutes tacked on to the end of your morning shower

Instructions:

◉ Once you've completed your normal showering duties, nudge the water temperature to as cold as you can stand.

◉ Take a few deep breaths under the cold water.

◉ Switch the water temperature back toward warm.

◉ Take a few breaths here and repeat, working up to the biggest variance in temperatures you can stand.

◉ If you can, end on a cold cycle. (If it's cold outside or in your bathroom, it's fine to end on warm.)

Modifications:

◉ If you're menstruating or pregnant, skip this treatment. It can be too stimulating during a time when your body is otherwise occupied.

◉ Stop the treatment if you become dizzy or start shivering uncontrollably.

Benefits:

◉ The hot and cold water therapy causes your blood vessels to rapidly constrict and dilate. This boost in circulation then revs your metabolism, your heart, and your overall energy level.

◉ It helps you wake up without the accompanying jitters of an extra-large dose of caffeine.

◉ This will leave you feeling alert and ready to face whatever trials the day may bring.

Other Remedies to Try:
A Filling and Energizing Breakfast
Invisible Trampoline • Ring the Gong

Lethargy

No matter how many things are going on in your life, nothing sounds as good to you as lying on the couch—you can't seem to find the initiative to do much of anything. Your listlessness is probably a clue from your body that it could use some good old-fashioned rest. Take a nap if you can, or go to bed early tonight—the more you heed your body's clues, the less you'll feel like you're swimming upstream. But, of course, time is always a precious commodity. If there's no room for a nap in your schedule, or if you've done plenty of resting and now need to get going, here's an exercise that can help you shake off inertia and reignite your inner fire in mere minutes. It comes from *qigong,* a system of exercise developed 3,000 years ago by Chinese peasants as a way to ward off physical and mental malaise. Built on the principle that everyone has an inherent supply of vital energy, or *qi* (pronounced "chee'), *qigong* ("chee gung," which translates as "energy work") aims to get the body moving in order to remove stagnant energy and usher in fresh, vibrant energy. This particular exercise is known as "Ring the Gong" because, as you move, your hands will lightly slap your torso, making you the gong in this scenario. And the ringing of a gong is a universal signal that it's time to wake up, snap to attention, and move on to the next thing. Prepare to kiss your couch goodbye. 🌸

Remedy:
Ring the Gong

Ingredients:
Three feet of clear floor space—enough to be able
to swing your arms out to your sides without hitting
anything

Time Needed:
One to two minutes

Instructions:
◉ Stand with feet several inches apart—about as wide as your shoulders—toes facing forward, arms dangling by your sides, knees bent slightly.

◉ Begin slowly twisting your body to the right and then to the left. Let your thighs, hips, belly, shoulders, neck, and head all get in on the action. Only your toes remain pointed forward.

🌀 Keep your arms soft as you move and let them rise and fall naturally as you twist.

🌀 Gradually build up the momentum so that you are twisting farther and faster. As you do, your arms will begin to rise up higher and lightly slap your rib cage as you reach the end of each twist.

🌀 Continue breathing smoothly through your nose as you move.

🌀 After approximately twenty rounds, begin slowing down your movement. You won't twist as far and your arms won't rise as high.

🌀 Gradually come back to a standstill in the starting position.

Modifications:

🌀 You can make the intensity as high or as low as you like by varying the speed of your twists. Doing it slowly is more meditative, while moving quickly is clearly more physical. Neither way is "right"—do what feels best to you and your body.

Benefits:

🌀 Twists the spine, which wrings tension out of your back and loosens things up so that energy can travel more freely around along this nervous system superhighway

🌀 Stimulates your abdominal organs, which spurs digestion and elimination

🌀 Encourages you to get up and get moving without requiring you to don special clothes, leave the house, or get all sweaty and red in the face

Other Remedies to Try:
Hot/Cold Water Therapy • Hot Ginger Tea
Invisible Trampoline • Plank Pose

PMS

You may be weepy, cranky, bloated, achy, or exhausted—or any combination of the above. Oh, the cruel hand of fate! There's nothing you can do except pop a Midol and bravely soldier on . . . right? Although there's no denying that a wicked bout of PMS is a definite challenge—sometimes even a debilitating one—there is another way to approach it.

Historically, a woman's period was a time of sanctioned rest. In Chinese medicine, menstrual blood is referred to as "heavenly water," whereas we are more likely to see it as a monthly curse. Chinese and Indian medicine revere the menstrual cycle because it gives women a chance to purge impurities—physical and mental—every month, and these traditions even believe that this relates to why women live longer than men. Although we've come a long way in equality between the sexes since ancient times, and our tampon commercials now flaunt women riding bikes and climbing mountains, perhaps we've lost some wisdom. I'm not suggesting that you take to your bed for a week each month as you sip broth and sniff vapors. But if you're suffering through a whammy of PMS every month, it may be a cry for help from your body, begging you to treat yourself more gently throughout your monthly cycle.

This restorative yoga pose is a fabulous way to do just that. It soothes your frazzled nerves, opens your chest and abdomen so you can breathe more deeply, and increases blood flow to the pelvis to reduce cramps and congestion. And best of all, it feels fantastic. Try doing it daily in the days leading up to and through your period. You can even do it once in the morning and once again before bed. Your husband or boyfriend might initially look at you a little funny, but if he's smart, he'll put it together pretty quickly that when you start dragging out the couch cushion, a little extra consideration from him will go a long way toward a happier you in the days ahead. It's just another benefit of taking good care of yourself—the more you do for yourself, the more the people around you will start doing for you, too. ✿

Remedy:
Supported Reclining Bound Angle Pose

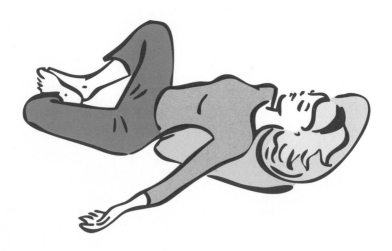

Ingredients:
A firm pillow or couch cushion
A thin blanket or towel, folded to
make a small square pillow

Time Needed:
Five minutes

Instructions:

◎ Place your cushion on the floor and the folded towel at one end of the cushion.

◎ Sit on the floor with your back grazing the empty edge of the cushion.

◎ Bring the soles of your feet to touch and allow your bent knees to fall out to the sides.

◎ Draw your heels in toward your pelvis.

◎ Lean back on to your hands and then proceed to lay your spine down on the cushion.

◎ Adjust the towel to support your head and neck (but not your shoulders). You want your forehead to be slightly higher than your chin so that the back of your neck stays nice and long.

◎ Once you're situated, rest your arms—palms facing up—on the floor a few inches away from your torso.

◎ Let yourself sink into the floor and the cushion as you breathe evenly through your nose.

◎ Release any physical effort and simply allow yourself to relax, open, and soften.

◎ To come out of the pose, use your hands to draw your knees together. Roll over into the fetal position on one side, and then press both of your hands palms down into the floor to push yourself back up to a seated position.

Modifications:

🌀 If you feel a stretch in your inner thighs that makes it difficult to rest comfortably for the full five minutes, place a rolled-up towel underneath each thigh.

🌀 If you experience tightness or any unpleasant sensation in your lower back when in the pose, pick up your pelvis, roll your sitting bones and buttocks toward your heels, and then lower your pelvis to the floor again. Start with only one minute in the pose, gradually working your way up to a longer time as your lower back allows. If neither of these adjustments relieves your lower back pain, this pose is not for you—see the remedy for cramps instead.

Benefits:

🌀 Opens the chest and encourages deeper breathing, which helps clear your mind and calm your nerves so that you can get off the emotional roller coaster

🌀 Relieves congestion and heaviness in the abdomen, reducing cramps and giving your body a little head start on the monthly cleaning it's about to begin

🌀 Gives you a way to consciously relax that also feels physically delicious—the perfect way to give yourself the TLC you're craving

Other Remedies to Try:
Supported Child's Pose
Supported Seated Forward Bend

Cramps

enstrual cramps are stealing a day or two away from your normal life each month, whether they're the sharp, piercing kind often accompanied by diarrhea or the type that feels more like a dull ache, complete with bloating, gas, and constipation. Either way, they're no walk in the park. Many women want only to curl up into a ball until they subside.

This yoga pose is a forward bend, and it shares that curling in on oneself quality with the fetal position. But this pose also opens up the entire back of the body and encourages blood and energy to circulate more freely to the abdomen and uterus, helping to flush this area and soothe its spasms. Because it allows you to put your head down and rest—like a cranky elementary school student in need of a little time-out—it also calms frazzled nerves and helps quiet your thoughts. It may not make all of your pain magically disappear, but it will help you move the needle toward feeling better so that you feel as if life is indeed manageable.

It also calms frazzled nerves and helps quiet your thoughts.

Remedy:
Supported Seated Forward Bend

Ingredients:
Wooden dining chair or metal folding chair

Time Needed:
Two to five minutes

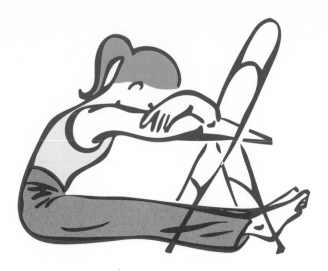

Instructions:

🌀 Sit on the floor (near the chair) with your legs outstretched in front of you.

🌀 Pick up the chair and place it over your legs so that the inner edge of the seat is perpendicular to the middle of your shin.

🌀 As you inhale, extend your arms over your head and let this lifting action lengthen your torso up away from the floor.

🌀 Exhale and bend forward at your hips. Cross your forearms and rest them on the chair seat and cushion your forehead on your top forearm.

🌀 Permit your back to be slightly rounded, but balance this action by concentrating on letting your spine be long and reaching forward, away from your hips.

🌀 Release any effort from your abdomen.

◎ Stay here, breathing deeply through your nose and allowing your head to sink into your arms, as long as it feels good, for up to five minutes.

Modifications:

◎ If this pose causes an intense and uncomfortable stretch in your back or in the back of your thighs, fold a blanket and slip it under your buttocks.

◎ Experiment with having your legs hips' distance apart and totally together, and go with whatever variation feels best to you.

◎ Skip this pose if you feel nauseated or are experiencing diarrhea. Try the remedy for PMS instead, which will also help with cramps.

Benefits:

◎ Brings an influx of fresh blood—and therefore oxygen— to the abdomen, which revitalizes the area and helps the organs there carry out their functions of digestion and reproduction (net result: cramps are alleviated)

◎ Stretches the hamstrings and the back, making you feel looser all over

◎ Allows the head and the mind to rest, alleviating irritability, anxiety, and headaches

---

Other Remedies to Try:
Hot Ginger Tea • Supported Child's Pose
Supported Reclining Bound Angle Pose

Cold

*Y*our head is throbbing, energy is zapped, and poor little nose is raw from all the blowing you've done. Although a cold can surely make you miserable, it isn't generally debilitating. Meaning you can't get all doped up on cold medicine because you still need to be able to take care of business. Even though you're likely still going to work, you do require some extra care—the kind that just doesn't come in pill form.

> *You do require some extra care—the kind that just doesn't come in pill form.*

While there are myriad remedies you can take, from echinacea and zinc to Alka-Seltzer Plus and cough syrup, the key components to getting over a cold are heaping helpings of fluids and rest. Here's a recipe for a delicious and soothing fluid to sip while you take it as easy as your schedule will allow. You can drink it at work or at home, and you can prepare it in mere minutes, making it the time-poor woman's version of homemade chicken soup. May it help you get back to your normal self quickly and ease the cold-related misery until you do. 🌸

Remedy:
Hot Water with Lemon and Honey

Ingredients:
Water
Honey
Fresh lemon

Time Needed:
Three minutes to prepare, several more to sip

Instructions:

🌀 Heat water as you would for tea—whether that's on the stovetop, in an electric kettle, or in the microwave.

🌀 When the water is steaming in your mug, swirl in a teaspoon or so of honey and a few squeezes of fresh lemon to taste.

🌀 Savor the sweet smells—if you can!—as you sip.

🌀 Repeat several times a day until the fog lifts.

Modifications:
N/A

Benefits:

🌀 The hot water breaks up phlegm and stimulates your digestion, which helps fight the sluggish feeling that often accompanies colds.

🌀 The lemon is astringent, which dries up mucus.

🌀 The honey has natural antiviral and antibacterial properties and is a good source of fructose, which provides energy that lasts longer than the kick you get from refined sugar.

Other Remedies to Try:
Hot Ginger Tea • Probiotics
Third Eye Acupressure

Eczema

verything was going along fine. Then the work began piling up on your desk, you ate a string of highly processed meals, tossed your way through a few sleepless nights, and boom— your recurring itchy, red rash suddenly burst into bloom, again.

A group nearly twice the size of New York City suffers from eczema, so if your outbreaks make you feel like a lone pariah, know that you are by no means alone. Although there is no known "cure," there are many things you can do to help yourself break out of the cycle of stress, breakout, embarrassment, and slow healing process.

Enter probiotics—friendly bacteria that colonize the digestive tract and perform three major functions: They produce vitamins and enzymes that help the body absorb more nutrients and more efficiently eliminate waste; keep harmful bacteria in check; and assist the immune system, with particular emphasis on preventing it from overreacting. Taking a probiotic supplement can go a long way toward avoiding future outbreaks. (See "Instructions" and "Benefits" for more information on why they work and how to take them.)

Eczema is often tied to allergies—in both instances, your immune system reacts to something it perceives as a threat. And your immune system and digestive system work in tandem—after all, the digestive system is how we first encounter foreign particles through food, drink, and air. When you find yourself experiencing frequent eczema flare-ups, prioritize good digestive health by eating ground flaxseeds (see the Constipation remedy for more information) in addition to taking probiotics. The seeds contain fiber, so they help keep your digestion humming. They are also a rich source of omega-3 fatty acids, which can help combat the inflammation and itchiness associated with eczema.

And finally, instead of noticing the first signs of an eczema outbreak and despairing, take it as a sign that you need to prioritize your self-care. Recurrent conditions such as eczema are your body's way of saying, "Hey, lady, could you take it easy, please?" Refer to the Overwhelmed entry for the instructions for Supported Child's Pose—a fabulous way to soothe your nervous system and support yourself during trying times—and do it every day until the attack subsides. ❧

> *Take it as a sign that you need to prioritize your self-care.*

Remedy:
Probiotics

Ingredients:

Probiotic supplements that contain *Lactobacillus rhamnosus GG*—a particular strain of friendly bacteria that studies suggest is an effective preventative measure for eczema

Time Needed:

Fifteen to thirty minutes to buy the supplements; seconds a day to take them

Instructions:

◎ Visit your health food store to buy the supplements. Probiotics will likely be kept in a refrigerated case since the cultures in the supplements are living microbes.

◎ Talk with one of the employees in the supplement section and find out if customers have reported a greater success with a particular brand.

◎ Check the expiration date and be sure that you'll be able to take all of the supplements before then.

◎ Keep the bottle in your refrigerator at home.

◎ Take one capsule a day during outbreaks or series of outbreaks.

◎ For best results, open the capsule and sprinkle the probiotics on a plate of cold or lukewarm food so that your mouth and esophagus—vital components of the digestive system—can be exposed to them. (Since the probiotics are living cultures, scorching hot food could kill them.)

Modifications:

◎ If you need to travel, don't worry. Many probiotic strains can live up to two weeks without refrigeration. Just pack your probiotic pills as you would any other vitamin and continue to take them while you're away.

◎ When you're experiencing an outbreak or series of outbreaks, prioritize taking a supplement pill. In between attacks, taking the pills a few times a week will help keep your bacterial ecosystem in balance.

◎ Food sources of probiotics include cultured foods such as yogurt and kefir and fermented foods such as sauerkraut, miso, kimchi, and tofu. Include more of these foods in your diet as well.

Benefits:

◎ Taking probiotics improves the ratio of good bacteria to bad in your digestive tract, which helps your body derive more nourishment from the food you eat and boosts your ability to process and remove waste from the body.

◎ A highly controlled study of breastfeeding mothers with an immediate relative or partner with a history of allergies, eczema, or asthma who consumed probiotic supplements for the first six months of their babies' lives found that those children were up to 50 percent less likely to develop eczema by the time they turned two. While probiotics won't instantly "cure" your eczema, studies do suggest that they can help your body function more efficiently, thereby mitigating future attacks.

◎ Other studies have shown that probiotics can increase elimination, reduce the severity and duration of colds, clear up diarrhea, improve the efficacy of flu shots—even decrease the risk of diabetes.

◎ While there are no harmful side effects associated with taking probiotics, if you notice an initial increase in flatulence and bloating, simply cut down your dosage and slowly build up to one capsule a day. This reaction is likely merely an indicator that the probiotics are doing their job and killing off a large number of not-so-friendly bacteria, which are producing an uptick in waste products as they die off.

Other Remedies to Try:
Ground Flaxseeds • Supported Child's Pose

Tight Back, Shoulder, or Neck Muscles

Oh, your aching back. Your shoulders have taken up permanent residence somewhere around your ears, your lower back is so tight you could bounce a quarter off it, or your neck yowls in pain when you turn it too quickly. And if you're at your worst, perhaps all three things are happening at once.

The back is a crucial player in your own personal support system. But because it's behind you and therefore out of your sight, most people rarely give it a second thought. Until it starts talking to you in little twinges, aches, or spasms, that is. Don't wait until your back has to start screaming to get your attention—as soon as you notice it's becoming tight, clear a little space on your floor, block off fifteen minutes in your schedule, and get busy giving yourself some love with the help of two cute, furry, yellow tennis balls. Yes, tennis balls. They are the perfect size and density to really work over the major muscles of the back (in a good way). And you can't beat the price—about $2 for three of them. ✿

Remedy:
Tennis Ball Massage

Ingredients:
Two tennis balls
Carpet, towel, or yoga mat to make the
floor comfortable enough to lie on
Folded blanket or firm pillow to support
your neck and shoulders

Time Needed:
Fifteen to twenty minutes

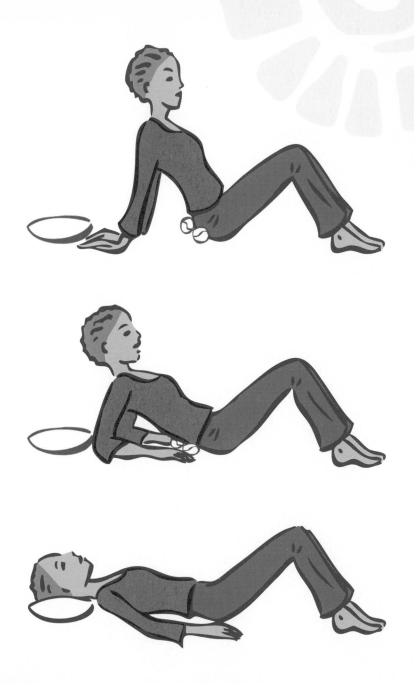

Instructions:

⊚ Sit on the floor with your legs bent and feet flat on the floor.

⊚ Place the two tennis balls on either side of your spine just behind you on the floor.

⊚ Place your palms on the floor behind you and, propping the weight of your torso on your hands, lift your seat up just enough to come to sit on the tennis balls. They should be on either side of your tail bone.

⊚ Take three to five breaths here, allowing the tennis balls to penetrate the muscles in your buttocks.

⊚ After three to five breaths, roll your hips toward your feet so the tennis balls move further up the lowest part of your back an inch or two.

⊚ Take several breaths here; then roll again. Keep working the balls up your spine this way.

⊚ When it feels comfortable to you, lower your elbows to the floor so that your arms don't have to overwork to keep your torso supported. The idea is to soften as much as possible at each step of the way.

⊚ Once the tennis balls reach the bottom of your rib cage, bring your torso all the way down and rest your head and neck on the folded-up blanket or firm pillow.

⊚ When you reach your neck, use your hands to keep the tennis balls from popping out to the side.

⊚ When you've massaged the entire spine, remove the tennis balls and the cushion from under your head and lie flat on the floor for a few breaths, noticing the difference in how your back feels from before you started.

Modifications:

◎ When you find a spot where the sensation of the tennis balls is particularly intense—and you will—either rock slowly so that the pressure isn't constant, or move the tennis balls slightly up or down until you find the point where you can tolerate the intensity.

Benefits:

◎ Spending several breaths working on each spot releases the stiffer connective tissue that holds the muscles in place as well as the muscles themselves.

◎ This increases blood flow to the back of your body, encouraging tension and stress to wash away as new energy rushes in.

◎ It offers a cheap, simple way to indulge yourself (no expensive trips to a fancy spa required—although fancy spas definitely have their time and place, you can't exactly go every week).

> **Other Remedies to Try:**
> Legs Up the Wall • Shoulder Bounces
> Supported Child's Pose
> Supported Seated Forward Bend
> Warrior 1 Pose

Aching Feet

You've been pounding the pavement in shoes that weren't meant to do much more than look sexy, and your poor feet are throbbing. Ease that ache with this simple (and free) massage technique that can be done while you watch TV, take a bath, or lie in bed. Yes, it looks a little funny. But when you're finished, your feet will feel so revived and relaxed, you won't care one whit what it looks like. ❀

Remedy:
Hold Hands with Your Feet

Ingredients:
One hand and one foot

Time Needed:
Four minutes—two for each foot

Instructions:

◎ Take off your shoes and socks, panty hose, or tights.

◎ Sit or lie down somewhere you can comfortably rest while holding one of your feet with your hands.

◎ When you've got a hold of your foot, work the fingers of the opposite hand in between your toes. Try to interweave your fingers all the way to the webbing. Be gentle—your toes likely haven't moved away from each other in quite some time. Move a little distance at a time and only work your fingers in deeper when your foot has had a chance to accommodate the stretch.

◎ Spend a few moments here simply breathing and imagining any tension in your feet dissipating with each exhale.

◎ Once you've grown used to the stretch, use your fingers to move your toes forward and backward and around in a circle.

◎ Then use your thumb to massage the ball and arch of your foot.

◎ After about two minutes, switch feet.

Modifications:

◎ If you have trouble working your fingers in, try a little hand lotion or foot cream. Although this exercise will likely produce a strong stretching sensation, back off or stop altogether if you feel any sharp pains.

Benefits:

◎ Stretches the muscles and ligaments of the front of the foot, which get especially stressed when wearing high heels

◎ Promotes flexibility in and creates space in between the toes, giving you a more supple and stable platform to stand upon

◎ Dramatically changes the way your feet feel—no expensive pedicure or foot massage required

◎ Offers you yet another way to take great care of yourself without a lot of time, accoutrements, or effort

> **Other Remedies to Try:**
> Legs Up the Wall

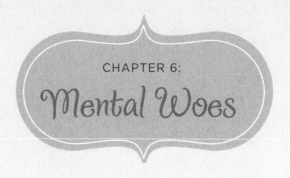

CHAPTER 6:

Mental Woes

When your mood tanks or thoughts start spiraling out of control, Western culture typically advocates that you A) give it time, B) talk to a professional, or C) take a prescription designed to alter your brain chemistry. While all of these tactics can be helpful and have their time and place, they aren't your sole options. You have plenty of tools at your disposal—your breath, your intention, and your body—to start moving the needle on your own mental and emotional well-being back toward balance.

You may have noticed that you feel more relaxed after a run, less irritable after a meal, or a little better about a vexing problem after a full night's sleep. These are all basic examples of how targeting the body also affects the mind. This chapter delves into do-it-yourself mental and emotional maintenance so that next time you find yourself roiling with anger, or fearful of an upcoming change, or in need of an attitude adjustment, you'll have some techniques in your back pocket that can help you navigate life's twists and turns with grace instead of grumpiness, patience instead of panic.

Angry

Someone has gone and done it now, whatever "it" may be, and you are seething. The anger has risen up to your eyeballs, and you're left wondering what to do to relieve some of the buildup. Anger is a powerful form of energy that needs to be released or it will fester and grow, like a boil that needs to be lanced. The good news is that you can, in fact, find a nonviolent way to vent those pent-up feelings, and you don't need to block out

You simply need to be willing to look a little silly and get up off your duff.

an hour or more of your day to go for a run or hit the gym. Nor does it require you to karate chop a two-by-four with your bare hands, or remain still and breathe—about the last thing you need at this very moment. You simply need to be willing to look a little silly and get up off your duff to do something you probably haven't done since elementary school: bounce.

Remedy:
Invisible Trampoline

Ingredients:
Privacy

Time Needed:
Two to five minutes

Instructions:
Stand with your feet several inches apart, knees slightly bent, and arms dangling by your sides.

◎ Begin bouncing up and down until your feet start lifting up off the floor.

◎ Hold your body as soft as possible to keep this a low-impact exercise—no locked knees, rigid arms, or motionless neck. Let your arms bounce along with you.

◎ With each jump, lift up off the ground as much (or as little) as you like.

◎ Once you've been at it awhile, jump in a full circle to your right and then to your left. You can also travel around the room if you like.

◎ Gradually slow your movements down before eventually coming to a complete stop.

Modifications:

◎ If you're comfortable, make some cathartic vocal noises while you jump. Whatever sound you choose to make, whether it's a primal scream or some well-chosen curse words, shout it with the intention of purging your anger, not adding to it.

◎ Listening to music as you jump makes it easier to really let yourself go and shake off whatever's bothering you.

◎ Anger is often an outward manifestation of a deeper fear or hurt. Once you've rid yourself of some of your excess energy, spend a little time tending to your heart with the remedy for depression (Supported Heart Opener).

Benefits:

◎ Gives you something constructive to do with the pent-up energy that's surging through your body

◎ Makes you look and feel silly—a good reminder of the levity in the world despite whatever has you so upset

◎ Shakes you out of your dark mental state

◎ Gets your blood flowing and brings a flush to your cheeks

Other Remedies to Try:
Chamomile Tea • Lion Pose in the Bathroom
Stimulate Your "Letting Go" Acupressure Point
Supported Heart Opener

Cranky

*E*very little thing is setting you off—the sound your boyfriend makes when he chews his food, the way the driver in front of you changes lanes without signaling, how someone moved your leftovers in the office fridge. You're spending so much time being annoyed, in fact, that you're starting to bug even yourself.

Although crankiness can seem as if it stems from plain ol' meanness, it's more likely that you're overtired, overworked, and/or overstressed. What you need is a simple way to soothe yourself. Then you'll be better able to forgive minor transgressions and view other people as your allies, not a source of irritation.

Although anger and crankiness are cousins, crankiness is a pebble in your shoe whereas anger is a boulder falling on your head. As such, the remedy for crankiness (sipping chamomile tea) is subtler than the remedy for anger (jumping up and down as if you were on an invisible trampoline). Chamomile is a flower widely hailed by herbalists and practitioners of Ayurveda—the ancient system of medicine from India—for its remarkable calming capabilities. Even Peter Rabbit's mother was hip to its charms—when Peter was chased by Mr. McGregor and came running home, nose quivering with panic, she fixed him a cup and sent him to bed.

In a moment of emotional upset, the real power of chamomile tea comes from inhaling its aroma. Smells take a shortcut to the brain and can help change your mood before your rational mind can even register exactly what it smells. Try it next time you need to calm down in a hurry. 🌸

Remedy:
Chamomile Tea

Ingredients:
Chamomile tea bags—the best quality you can find

Time Needed:
Three minutes to prepare the tea, five to ten minutes to savor

Instructions:
🌀 Unwrap a tea bag and place it in an empty mug.

🌀 Boil water.

🌀 Fill the mug with hot water.

🌀 As the tea steeps, hold the mug in your hands and take big whiffs of the floral aroma. Really get your nose down in there and breathe deeply.

🌀 Notice the sensation of warmth in your hands and the way it travels through your nose as you inhale. Keep your mind focused solely on the act of drinking tea—no watching TV, checking your e-mail, or talking on the phone allowed.

🌀 Slowly sip the tea as you continue to enjoy the scent.

🌀 There, there—isn't that better?

Modifications:

🌀 If you don't have time for the whole tea-making ritual, you can also buy chamomile essential oil at your health food store and keep it in your purse or desk drawer. When you feel your irritation welling up, uncap the bottle and take a few deep breaths until you feel soothed.

🌀 Or, if you want to step your soothing up a notch, add a few drops of chamomile essential oil or several chamomile tea bags to a warm bath.

Benefits:

🌀 Chamomile soothes the nervous system and eases stress, anxiety, and nervous disorders.

🌀 It is also a powerful tonic to the digestive system and can soothe an upset stomach.

Other Remedies to Try:
Belly Breathing
Mini Loving Kindness Meditation
Supported Child's Pose

Stressed

You have so many things going on that it takes every bit of energy just to make it through your daily list of must-dos. And you can tell the frantic pace is starting to take its toll because your temper is flaring, you're sleeping less, and you seem to be catching every bug that crosses your path. Stress has sunk its teeth into you.

> It takes every bit of energy just to make it through your daily list of must-dos.

Luckily, you don't have to book a week at a spa or steal away for a tropical vacation to start extricating yourself from stress's grip. (Although, clearly, these are lovely options and highly recommended if they are available to you.) You can start right here, right now, in this very moment, simply by taking a big ol' breath. Your diaphragm—the parachute-shaped muscle that extends across the bottom of your rib cage—is a key player in your body's reaction to stress. When you hold your breath or breathe shallowly—a typical reaction to a stressful situation—your diaphragm doesn't get a chance to expand. And when the diaphragm is locked up, it sends a message to the rest of your body that there is danger afoot and you had best start preparing for the worst. But when you take a long, slow breath down into your belly, your diaphragm inflates downward like a balloon, creating more room for your lungs to expand, gently pressing down on and massaging your abdominal organs, and telling the rest of your body that everything is okay.

By pausing to take even one deep breath, you also give yourself a chance to reflect before you react so you're less likely to do something that only creates more stress in your life. And the more you do it, the more you'll relax and become better able to roll with life's punches instead of taking them on the chin. ❀

Remedy:
Belly Breathing

Ingredients:
Lungs
Belly
Hands

Time Needed:
Anywhere between ten seconds and ten minutes

Instructions:

◉ Sit up tall in your chair and place both feet flat on the floor.

◉ Rest one or both hands on your stomach, just below your navel.

◉ Inhale through your nose. As you do, imagine sending your breath deep into your belly. You'll know you're doing it right because the hand that is resting on your belly will move away from your spine as you inhale. Take in as much air as you can.

◉ Allow the breath to seep slowly out through your nostrils as you feel your belly deflate and your hand move back in toward your spine.

◉ Repeat until you feel better.

Modifications:

◉ If you have more time, try the exercise lying down on the floor with a thin pillow under your head and a rolled-up blanket or towel under your knees. By not having to work to hold yourself upright, you'll be able to give yourself over even more to the relaxing effects of the practice.

⊚ Even if you are in the middle of an insane day and can't set aside even one minute to focus solely on your breathing, you can take one deep belly breath and repeat on an as-needed basis. You can do it surreptitiously while on the phone, in a meeting, driving your car, or even walking down the street.

⊚ You don't *have* to place your hand on your stomach—it merely gives you a physical point of reference to help make the exercise more tactile. If it embarrasses you or you forget, don't sweat it.

Benefits:

⊚ Triggers your relaxation response

⊚ Invites more oxygen into and flushes more waste products out of the lungs, helping the body work more efficiently

⊚ Massages the abdominal organs and improves digestion

⊚ Promotes better sleep when done regularly

⊚ Gives your mind something to focus on other than whatever's causing you stress, even if only for a moment

Other Remedies to Try:
Center of Power Stimulation
Chamomile Tea• Rescue Remedy
Sphinx Pose
Stimulate Your "Letting Go" Acupressure Point

Scattered

There's so much going on in your life that at any given moment, you're not sure what to do with yourself. Work duties, your e-mail inbox, your list of calls that need to be returned—it sometimes feels like so much is demanding your attention that your ability to focus has all but disappeared, leaving you with piles of half-finished products and a never-ending sense that there's at least ten things you should be doing right now. If only you could decide which task is most important, perhaps you could actually work your way down the list.

In today's go-go-go world, it's perfectly understandable to feel like you're stuck on a treadmill that's moving too fast with no off button. Take your stress levels down a notch and increase your focus by taking a few minutes to apply pressure to the acupuncture point directly in the center of the space between your eyebrows—otherwise known as your third eye. Tapping into this all-important point quickly calms the nervous system and the mind so that you can concentrate. Yogis also believe that your third eye is the seat of your intuition. According to this perspective, stimulating your third eye will allow you to access your inner wisdom to decide where your efforts are most needed instead of letting outside pressure or panic lead the way.

> *You're stuck on a treadmill that's moving too fast with no off button.*

Remedy:
Third Eye Acupressure

Ingredients:
Fingertips

Time Needed:

One to two minutes

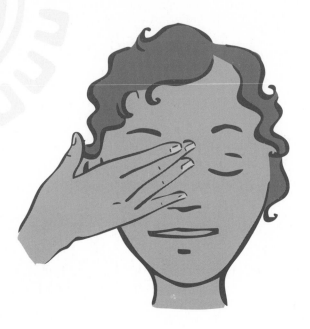

Instructions:

🌀 Sit up tall in your chair with the soles of both feet fully on the floor.

🌀 Locate the slight indentation at the spot in between your eyebrows where the bridge of your nose meets your forehead.

🌀 Use one of your middle fingers to apply firm pressure to the spot as you breathe deeply. Because you're trying to promote focus, close your eyes to turn your attention inward instead of letting your gaze dart around the room.

◉ After ten to fifteen deep breaths, gradually release the pressure and allow your breathing to return to normal.

◉ Let both hands rest in your lap and briefly visualize yourself performing your next task with ease and efficiency before diving back into your to-do list.

Modifications:

◉ If you're in need of a more serious dose of grounding and relaxation, bring your palms to touch in front of your chest, then lift your hands so that the tips of both middle fingers are pressing on your third eye point. This simple hand gesture signifies surrender, although it is a little more likely to get people around you wondering what in the heck you're doing. Let your need and your surroundings guide you as you decide how to apply your pressure. And be careful if you have long nails.

Benefits:

◉ Calms the mind, reducing anxiety and confusion and promoting clearer, calmer thinking

◉ Also used in acupressure to relieve headaches, insomnia, and sinus congestion

Other Remedies to Try:
One-Minute Visualization
Supported Child's Pose
Swim in Your Own Sea of Tranquility

Overwhelmed

*E*verybody needs something from you and they need it *now*. Life is coming at you so fast, it feels like you've been knocked under water by a large wave and you don't know which way is up. Where oh where is your fairy godmother when you need her?

Give yourself the solace you're craving with a supported child's pose. It's profoundly relaxing, feels absolutely divine, and you can do it as much as you like until you feel replenished and ready to meet your challenges head on.

Remedy:
Supported Child's Pose

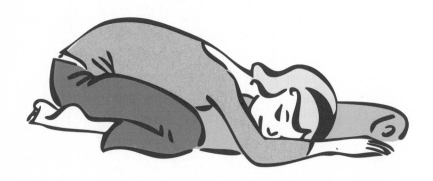

Ingredients:
Three feet of floor space cushioned with carpet, blanket, or a yoga mat folded in half
Firm cushion, two folded blankets, or a yoga bolster

Time Needed:
Five to ten minutes

Instructions:

◎ Sit on the floor on your shins with your seat resting on your feet.

◎ Open your knees wide and place your cushion between your knees.

◎ Fold forward, bending at your hips, and rest your torso on the cushion.

◎ Turn your head to one side.

◎ Rest your arms either back by your hips, out to your sides, or crossed above your head and resting on the cushion—whatever feels most restful to you.

◎ Breathe here and give your body permission to fully relax.

◎ About halfway through your time in this pose, turn your head to the other side.

◎ Stay as long as it feels good to you.

◎ Slowly push yourself back to the starting position and rest a few breaths there before bounding off to your next task.

Modifications:

◎ If your knees are uncomfortable, roll up a hand towel or washcloth into a thin bundle and place it at the top of your calves just inside the creases at the back of your knees. This creates a little more space in the knee joint and should make the pose more tolerable for you.

◎ If your seat doesn't rest on your feet, either make the cushion under your chest taller or fold up another blanket and place it on top of your heels so your booty can rest.

Benefits:

◎ Calms the nervous system and quiets the mind, helping you think more clearly and shifting you out of anxiety mode

◎ Releases back and neck tension, giving you the sensation of shedding whatever burdens you may be carrying

◎ Also stretches the ankles, shins, and hips

◎ Having the cushion pressing into your abdomen also reduces cramps, making this a great pose to do when you have your period.

> **Other Remedies to Try:**
> Belly Breathing • Chamomile Tea
> Head Down Time Out

Afraid

*L*ife is requiring you to move outside of your comfort zone, and you're getting a funny, heavy feeling deep down in your stomach whenever you think about what's in store for you, whether it's public speaking, confronting a friend you're angry with, or starting a new job. That's fear making its presence known, and one of the best ways to usher it along is to open the hips.

Why the hips? That area of the body houses your first and second chakras. The first chakra is located at your tailbone—which you're sitting on right now—and rules survival. If you're scared that you won't be able to make rent this month or find a job that pays the bills, for example, that fear will probably settle at the very base of your pelvis. The second chakra rests just above the pubic bone, and it rules sexuality, emotions, creativity, and your ability to enjoy life. Feeling emotions, doing something creative, and opening yourself up to true intimacy with someone else can be scary propositions. So whether your fears are about practical concerns or emotional ones, they have most likely settled in your hips.

> Whether your fears are about practical concerns or emotional ones, they have most likely settled in your hips.

To top all that off, pretty much everyone in North America has tight hips because we spend so much time sitting in chairs with our hips closed off. The ball-and-socket hip joint has a huge range of motion—think about a roundhouse kick—that we generally don't access. If you were the Tin Man, your hips would be in need of a few squirts from the oilcan.

Luckily, there's an easy way to get some new blood, literally, flowing into the hips. A squat opens the whole hip area and flushes away anything that has grown stale and constricted. Squatting is like purging your closets—you're getting rid of stuff you don't need, don't use, don't have room for, and probably don't even like anymore. And as you're opening your hips, you're also opening yourself to new possibilities. If you're still skeptical that this is the pose for you, consider that women used to give birth while squatting—a testament to the pose's power to help the body usher in a new phase of life. Get ready to get empowered! ✿

Remedy:
Squat

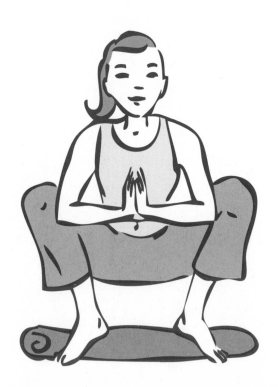

Ingredients:
Stretchy pants
Rolled-up towel (optional)
A wall (optional)

Time Needed:
One to two minutes

Instructions:

◎ Stand with your feet two to three feet apart, toes turned out slightly.

◎ Bend your knees deeply and lower your booty down toward the floor.

◎ Bring your palms together and rest your elbows on the insides of your knees. Use the leverage of your elbows gently pressing into your knees to lift your spine up taller and create more space for your chest to broaden.

◎ Lift the top of your head up toward the sky as your tail-bone descends toward the floor.

◎ Take five to ten slow, deep breaths. Imagine your inhales swirling around your hip joints and your exhales sweeping away any tension or constriction.

◎ To return to standing, press the soles of your feet firmly into the floor and straighten your legs.

◎ Because your hips are likely pretty creaky, repeat at least once to promote further opening.

Modifications:

⊚ If your heels rise up off the floor when you squat down, place a rolled-up towel underneath them. You want to feel grounded and secure as you invite your fears and hesitations to move along, so if your feet don't reach the ground, raise the ground up to meet you.

⊚ If the pose is too challenging overall, stand with your back a few inches away from a wall and let your back rest on the wall as you squat. And/or place a stack of phone books, magazines, or a yoga block under your booty and let your body weight rest on your support. There's no shame in using props.

⊚ Don't do this exercise if you're pregnant (unless you're working with a teacher or midwife or other alternative health practitioner who recommends it). Your ligaments are loosening to get ready for the baby, and you don't want to get too loose too early.

Benefits:

⊚ Opens the hips, pelvis, and lower back—the seat of your first and second chakras

⊚ Tones the abdomen, home to the third chakra—the source of your personal power, further empowering you to face your fears

⊚ Also provides a nice stretch for your ankles, making you better able to remain stable when the road gets bumpy

Other Remedies to Try:
Listen to Your Body • Rescue Remedy
Supported Child's Pose • Warrior's Breath

Depressed

Everyone gets the blues from time to time, when nothing seems to excite you or move you in any way, except to tears. Depression can be hormonal, only sticking around for a few days each month, or it can be a chronic case that unpacks its bags and decides to stay awhile. Although no one pose or practice can rectify all of your problems, this simple restorative yoga pose can create an opening in your body that in turn ushers in a more hopeful state of mind. When you feel the blues coming on, start practicing it every day. The combination of your intention and your action will help move the needle on your personal well-being gauge back toward happiness.

This supportive, heart-opening pose requires very little effort and feels great. It targets the chest, because the chest is the home of the heart. When you carry yourself with rounded shoulders, a hanging head, and a caved-in chest, you're cutting off the flow of blood and vitality to your physical and metaphorical heart. This easy pose gently stretches the area around the heart and invites fresh blood, oxygen, and vitality to flow in. Treat yourself whenever you need a pick-me-up. (It's a lot cheaper than retail therapy.) ❁

Remedy:
Supported Heart Opener

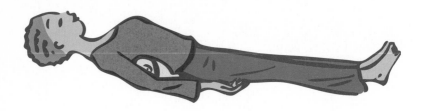

Ingredients:
Thin blanket or towel, rolled up in a tidy bundle
at least eighteen inches long

Time Needed:
Five to ten minutes

Instructions:

◎ Place your rolled-up towel or blanket on the floor.

◎ Sit with your back perpendicular to the blanket and your buttocks about two feet away.

◎ Lean back onto your elbows and gradually lower yourself to the floor. You ultimately want to be lying on the floor with the towel or blanket directly underneath your shoulder blades so that your heart is the highest point on the front of your body.

◎ Extend your legs and rest your arms on the floor by your sides with your palms facing up.

🌀 Lie here and breathe for up to ten minutes. Allow the weight of your body to sink farther and farther into the floor and the blanket.

🌀 Stay focused on your breath—now is not the time to brainstorm your grocery list or decide what to wear tomorrow.

🌀 When you're ready to come out, bend your knees and bring the soles of your feet to the floor. Roll on to your right side and rest in the fetal position for a moment before using your hands to push yourself up into a seated position.

Modifications:

🌀 Experiment with the thickness of your roll to find the height that feels best to you. Although you want to be comfortable, you do want to create a noticeable difference. So you don't want to be *too* comfortable.

🌀 You can also use a folded towel or blanket to support your head and shoulders if they don't quite reach the floor. Take care to make sure that your heart remains the highest point on your body.

Benefits:

🌀 Invites your metaphorical heart to bloom open, by physically creating space around your heart

🌀 Deepens your breathing, which triggers your relaxation response, stimulates your abdominal organs, invites more oxygen into the body, and generally makes you feel good all over

◎ Gives you a concrete way to do something nice for yourself at a time when you could use a little extra TLC

Other Remedies to Try:
Arms Up, Chest Up • Ground Flaxseeds • Self-Massage • Sphinx Pose
Warrior's Breath

Guilty

You have a heavy feeling in your chest that never completely fades, and it's because of something you did (or didn't do). That sensation is guilt making its presence known, and once it arrives, it's difficult to encourage it to move on unless you make a conscious effort to forgive yourself for whatever you've done.

This meditation technique gives you an opportunity to relive your actions and then forgive yourself for them. It aims to help you cultivate what Tibetan Buddhists call *metta* (or "loving kindness") toward yourself. It feels a heck of a lot better than constantly berating yourself, and it allows you to build your ability to feel compassion for yourself, which ultimately enables you to extend those same good feelings to everyone you encounter. You may not feel completely absolved after one session of loving kindness meditation. But keep practicing it, and notice as your mood and that lead apron on your chest start to lift. ❁

Remedy:
Loving Kindness Meditation (Toward Yourself)

Ingredients:
Whatever you need to sit comfortably with your spine tall—a firm cushion or folded blanket to sit on if you're using the floor, or a hard-backed chair

Time Needed:
Five to ten minutes

Instructions:

- Sit cross-legged with your booty resting on a cushion on the floor, or on the edge of a wooden chair with both feet flat on the floor.

- Rest your hands, palms up, on your thighs.

- Breathing through your nose, spend a few moments listening to the sound of your own breath and feeling the air moving in and out of your lungs.

- Once you've settled into a quieter state of mind, call up an image of yourself doing whatever it is that's now causing you guilt.

- With this picture in your mind, begin silently repeating, "I forgive myself for _____." Repeat several times. You can keep adding more things you forgive yourself for, or repeat one particular thing several times so it has a chance to sink in.

As you do this, notice any physical sensations. Do you feel a heaviness in your chest or stomach? A tightness in your jaw? Imagine releasing any negativity that arises with each exhale and inviting fresh new energy in as you inhale.

After you've worked through the situation in your mind, spend several breaths repeating a phrase such as "May I be happy, healthy, and free"—anything that expresses good wishes for yourself. If this phrase feels strange to you for any reason, choose another one that feels right to you. It could be "Bless my heart," "Grant me the serenity to accept the things I cannot change," or even "Amen."

When you feel done (and only you will know when that time is), return to simply listening to your breath for a few moments to give yourself a chance to absorb any emotional shifts you have just brought about.

Modifications:

If you become distracted by the physical effort to sit up straight, sit with your back resting on a wall or scoot back in your wooden chair so that the backrest supports your spine.

Keep your eyes open or closed, whichever feels most comfortable to you and appropriate to your surroundings.

You can also use this practice toward people who are working your nerves or causing you pain. But keep in mind that if you can't forgive yourself for your own perceived failings, it will be much harder to forgive others for theirs.

Benefits:

◎ This meditation builds your compassion muscles—an essential building block of forgiveness. Although this exercise focuses on you, it will also help you be more empathetic toward the difficult people in your life.

◎ It gives you an opportunity to own up to the things about yourself that you might like to change and invites them to move along.

◎ Meditating provides a tangible action you can do when you might otherwise be prone to sitting and stewing, which only makes you feel worse.

◎ Finally, it promotes relaxation and feelings of well-being at a time when you are feeling pretty down on yourself.

Other Remedies to Try:
Self-Massage • Supported Child's Pose
Warrior's Breath

Grieving

rief is an inevitable part of life, and about the only advice we ever receive is to "give it time"—essentially meaning, "ignore it and it will eventually fade." It's a natural tendency to want to avoid feelings of grief because they can be so painful. But the practice I suggest encourages those painful feelings to rise up so that they may ultimately lift completely.

This breathing exercise comes from yoga and can be done every day until you start to feel like yourself again. It's known as Warrior's Breath, and it invites fresh breath deep into the lungs where yoga and Chinese medicine believe grief takes up residence in the body. This belief makes sense from a practical standpoint—think about the last time you were so sad that you not only started crying, but your breath also got caught in your lungs, resulting in sobs. By filling this area with breath, you'll flush out any air or emotions that may have become lodged deep within the body and pave the way for new, more life-sustaining air to take its place.

> Encourage those painful feelings to rise up so that they may ultimately lift completely.

Don't discount the power of this exercise because it seems too simple—after you've done it for a minute or so, you'll realize that it takes all of your concentration and a considerable physical effort to keep going. Keep at it as long as you can, and if it elicits tears, don't be surprised. Just take them as a sign that your body is processing the grief, and notice how much better you feel when the tears are through. You're going to get through this, particularly now that you have something you can do to help the process along besides sitting around and waiting.

Remedy:
Warrior's Breath

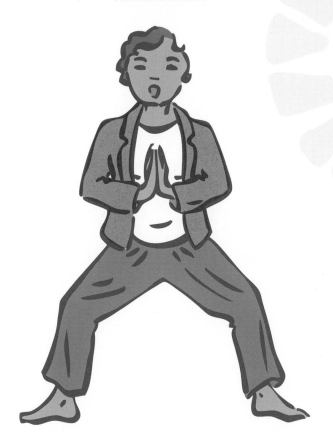

Ingredients:
Comfortable clothing
Bare feet

Time Needed:
Five to ten minutes

Instructions:

- Stand with your feet three to four feet apart, toes pointed out slightly.

- Bend your knees and lower your tush as if you were straddling an invisible horse.

- Bring your palms to touch in front of your heart.

- Inhale a deep breath through your nose as you reach your arms out to your sides at shoulder height, palms facing away from you.

- Exhale through your mouth, making a soft "ha" sound as if you were trying to fog up a mirror, as you bring your palms together again in front of your chest. Keep going.

- After you've got the hang of timing your movement to your breath and making the fog-up-a-mirror sound, begin exhaling through your nose while still making a similar "whoosh" noise. The noise won't be as loud, but it should still be audible to you.

- Continue as long as you can. Aim for at least fifteen breaths, more if you can hack it.

- When you're done, straighten your legs, bring your hands to your hips, and breathe normally for several moments before resuming normal activity.

Modifications:

- If standing with knees bent is too strenuous, you can also do this exercise while sitting cross-legged on the floor or on the edge of a hard-backed chair.

Benefits:

◎ The Warrior's Breath flushes stale air and old, stagnant emotions out of the lungs and torso.

◎ It bathes the lungs in fresh oxygen and energy.

◎ Making the "ha" sound requires that you constrict the back of your throat, which regulates the flow of air and adds a layer of mental complexity that gives you something to focus on other than how sad you are.

Other Remedies to Try:
Heart Meditation • Sphinx Pose
Supported Child's Pose
Supported Heart Opener

Anxious

Instead of eagerly anticipating future events, you're working yourself into a tizzy by imagining various worst-case scenarios. You're so busy churning away in your mind that it's starting to feel like there's no energy left for simple pleasures. Blech. You know that there must be a better way.

According to Chinese medicine, there are acupressure points on the outer chest known as "Letting Go." Stimulating these points balances the emotions by reducing tension in the chest and encouraging deep breathing. When you notice your thoughts spiraling out of control, spend a few minutes pressing these points per the following instructions to find your way back to more emotionally stable ground. ✿

Remedy:
Stimulate Your "Letting Go" Acupressure Point

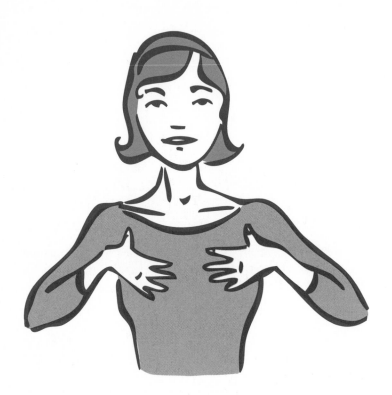

Ingredients:

Thumbs

Time Needed:

Two to three minutes

Instructions:

◉ Locate your Letting Go points by first finding your collarbones. They start at the bony points just below the hollow of your throat. Follow the bones out toward your shoulders. Letting Go is located on either side of your chest, three finger widths below the outer edges of the collarbones, in line with the inner edge of your armpits.

◉ Press your thumbs into the Letting Go points, applying pressure that is a combination of gentle and firm.

◉ Breathe deeply as you continue pressing these points for three minutes.

◉ Release the pressure gradually.

Modifications:

◉ Keep your eyes open or close them, depending on your surroundings and which is more soothing to you.

Benefits:

◉ Comforts your emotions, helping you to stop engaging in the thoughts that trigger anxiety

◉ Relieves muscle tension in the chest, paving the way for deeper breathing and, therefore, relaxation

◉ Also good for asthma

Other Remedies to Try:
Belly Breathing • Invisible Trampoline
Supported Child's Pose

Indecisive

Having the ability to make choices is one of the distinguishing benefits of being an adult. Babies don't get to decide when to have their diaper changed. Even teens don't get to say how long they'll stay out at night. But you, you can choose which job to take, where to live, who you want to hang out with, and whether you want to have Indian or Chinese for dinner. Sadly, even though being the master of your own fate is a privilege, making a decision often isn't easy. Whether you're pondering your next career move or trying to figure out what to wear, weighing your options and committing to a decision can become so mind-boggling that you almost wish someone would just tell you what to do.

> Even though being the master of your own fate is a privilege, making a decision often isn't easy.

To that end, you've asked your friends, your mom, the guy on the bus next to you this morning, and your Magic 8 ball—twice—for their opinions. Although other people's insights can be extremely valuable, the truth is, you're the only one who knows what's best for you. There's only one place left to turn. And that's inward. It's time to ask the wisest, most levelheaded part of yourself. Whether you call it a gut instinct, a hunch, or a feeling in your bones, everyone has an inner wisdom that resides deep within the body. This voice knows you better than anyone and always has a clear opinion about what you should do next. Unfortunately, it can't write urgent memos or leave a high-priority voice mail. For the most part, this voice speaks in physical sensations—a funny little tingle in your chest or an unexplained heavy feeling in your stomach, for instance—that you likely don't have time to notice, much less listen to. Today is the day that begins to change. . . .

Taking a few minutes to mentally check in with your body can help you make better decisions—the kind that seem to effortlessly result in a much happier you. It may feel like an exercise you really don't have time for, but consider how many hours spent making pro and con lists and lying awake at night pondering your future you could save. Best of all, the more you use this exercise, the better you'll get at it. With practice, you'll be able to access your inner wisdom in a matter of seconds simply by standing still and noticing what's going on in your body. Hey, it's a lot cheaper than the Psychic Friends Network. ✿

Remedy:
Listen to Your Body

Ingredients:
Someplace relatively quiet—a conference room, your parked car, even a public restroom

Time Needed:
Five minutes (and even less once you get better at hearing what your body has to say)

Instructions:
◉ Sit comfortably in your chosen spot.

◉ Turn off any distractions, such as the TV, your cell phone, or the computer.

◉ Inhale a deep breath and exhale out every last drop of air. Take three breaths this way to cue your body's relaxation response.

◎ Close your eyes if it helps you to relax and concentrate. If it only makes you feel sleepy, keep them open.

◎ Ask yourself the question you're wrestling with. *Should I find a new apartment? Is this the right guy/option for me?*

◎ Your job now is to notice:

◎ What's happening with your breath? Breathing shallowly, like a panting dog, is a sure sign of stress. Holding your breath can indicate fear. Slow, deep breaths point toward acceptance.

◎ How does your stomach feel? Does it feel heavy, like you swallowed a brick? Probably not a good sign. Is there a tingling there, or a lightness? This could indicate that some deeper part of you is truly excited about the proposition before you.

◎ How does your heart feel? As with your stomach, feeling heaviness is most likely a sign that the choice you're considering is not the best one for you. (You've heard the term "a heavy heart." It's pretty much universally considered something you don't want to have.) On the other hand, feeling warm or tingly points toward the fact that your metaphorical heart is with you on this one.

◎ Before you finish, scan your head, neck, shoulders, hips, legs, and feet. Any noteworthy sensation there, such as tightness (which can indicate stress) or tingling (which points toward excitement)?

◎ Open your eyes and take one more deep inhale and exhale to give yourself the chance to reacclimate to your surroundings before you go bounding off back into your day.

Modifications:

◉ Different people get messages from their inner wisdom in different ways. If you're listening to your body but it's not saying anything that you can understand, try writing down whatever comes to your mind. You don't have to have a special journal—scribbles on a legal pad work quite nicely.

◉ Or you may need movement to help quiet your mind. Try the exercise described above while walking, knitting, weeding, sweeping, or any other methodical activity that doesn't require your full concentration. Please don't try it while you're driving or chopping vegetables—some things really are best left to the rational mind.

◉ And if you try and don't hear anything, try again tomorrow. The more you do this, the better you'll get. It's just like learning to speak any new language. It takes time, patience, and practice.

◉ Finally, there are two types of fear. One is your body's way of alerting you that something isn't right and the situation may become dangerous. The other merely signals that you are moving out of your comfort zone—something every single one of us needs to do from time to time, scary as it may be, to keep moving forward. In my experience, the fear that signals danger feels heavier, like dread, while the other kind of fear has a lighter quality, like butterflies in your stomach—it might be the most intense case of butterflies you've ever had, but there is still a fluttery quality. As you become better at listening to your body, notice your own cues for each type of fear so that you can tell the difference between them.

This exercise is also particularly helpful in navigating the physical and emotional changes that accompany pregnancy. Developing a daily habit of checking in with your body to see what it needs to feel its best can help you ward off the nausea, fatigue, headaches, and mood swings that many women experience when they are carrying a baby.

Benefits:

Helps you stop obsessing and start taking action

Reduces your stress levels by helping you get out of limbo (otherwise known as purgatory)

Boosts your confidence in the choices you make (Guts don't lie.)

Sets the stage for you to sleep better, since you won't have to stay awake and ponder your future anymore

---

Other Remedies to Try:
Cobra Pose • Third Eye Acupressure

Forgetful

*L*ately you've been leaving home without your wallet, missing appointments, and completely forgetting to call people back. This has gone beyond your basic frazzled feeling and started making you wonder if you're going to end up being the youngest person ever diagnosed with Alzheimer's.

There are many reasons why you may be feeling this way: constantly feeling stressed, not getting enough sleep, and a typical American diet that's low in vital nutrients can all take their toll on your brain power. And, sadly, some cognitive decline is a natural part of the aging process. The key is to balance the parts of your life that drain your mental batteries with some simple practices that build it back up.

This technique helps combat stress and exhaustion, and it is so simple, even a third grader can do it. In fact, most of the people who do it are third graders. Remember in elementary school when the class would get too rowdy and your teacher would quiet things down by ordering the students to put their heads down on their desks? This is the exact same technique, coupled with a few basic alignment tips from yoga. You can do it at work or at home, even in the car (as long as you're parked, of course). It helps build mini mental vacations into your day so that you can calm down, rest your tired mind, and emerge feeling revitalized. Do it before meetings, starting a project, heading to the grocery store—anytime you need to think clearly.

For more mental measures, see the Modifications section of this remedy. 🌸

Remedy:
Head Down Time Out

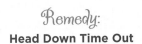

Ingredients:
Desk or table
Chair

Time Needed:
Two to three minutes

Instructions:

⊚ Sit in a chair facing a desk or table. Scoot your chair back about two feet from the edge of the desk.

⊚ Place both feet flat on the floor.

⊚ Fold at your hips and place your crossed forearms on the edge of your desk.

⊚ Rest your head on your forearms. Look straight down so the back of your neck is long and not wrenched in any one direction.

⊚ Reach your sit bones back so that your spine extends to its full length. The sides of your body, your back, and your abdomen should all feel like they're getting a nice stretch. (You may have to adjust the placement of your chair to allow for full extension.)

⊚ Close your eyes and breathe normally through your nose. Concentrate on releasing any tension you may be feeling with each exhale and inhaling new, revitalizing energy with each inhale.

⊚ Fully release the weight of your head into your forearms.

⊚ After two to three minutes, slowly come back to sitting up tall. Sit quietly for a few moments before resuming normal activity.

Modifications:

◎ Fuzzy thinking is often associated with an estrogen imbalance. The Chinese herb *dong quai* can help regulate estrogen levels whether you have too much or too little estrogen coursing through your veins. If your forgetfulness is chronic, speak with your chiropractor, doctor, acupuncturist, or other health care provider about an appropriate dosage for you. *Note:* Don't take *dong quai* if you have heavy periods, because it can instigate further bleeding.

◎ Omega-3 fatty acids are another supplement you should consider adding to your daily routine. Good sources include ground flaxseeds, flaxseed oil, oily fish such as salmon, and high-quality fish oil supplements. Omega-3's anti-inflammatory and mood-elevating properties are believed to promote better brain function.

◎ Not getting enough sleep also affects your ability to think clearly. If you're becoming noticeably more forgetful, prioritize your eight hours per night.

Benefits:

◎ Resting your head helps your brain shift off overload so that it can function more efficiently. It also quiets the nervous system so that you have more resources available for clear thinking.

◎ The mild shoulder and neck stretch removes tension from the area that serves as a bridge between mind and body, further allowing your thoughts to reach their destination.

◎ Finally, it builds a little rest into your day. While nothing beats getting more sleep, resting for a few minutes here and there can help refresh your mind and body.

> **Other Remedies to Try:**
> Arms Up, Chest Up • Supported Child's Pose
> Third Eye Acupressure

Stuck in a Rut

art of you is craving new experiences and stimulation, but the rest of you has its sights set firmly on wearing a groove in your daily routine—eating the same breakfast, taking the same route to work, hanging out with the same people, and watching the same shows. You want to mix it up, really you do, but maybe later when you're feeling a little more energized and focused and a little less afraid.

You can help usher in change instead of just waiting for it to arrive at your door by doing Plank Pose on a regular basis. It's incredibly heating, tones the whole body, builds your internal fire, and gives you the stamina and strength you need to go out there and shake things up. It also teaches you how to balance effort and surrender; because the pose is challenging, at some point you will have to go on faith that you can make it a little longer, just as you will need a balance of determination and trust to usher in the next phase of your life. ❧

Remedy:
Plank Pose

Ingredients:
Bare feet
Non-slidy surface, such as a hardwood floor
or a yoga mat

Time Needed:
One to two minutes

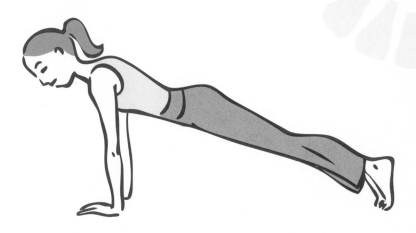

Instructions:

- Start on your hands and knees with your hands directly under your shoulders and your knees under your hips.

- Step both feet all the way back into the top of a push-up position. If you could see yourself from the side, you'd want to see one even line—be sure not to let your hips sag down toward the floor or rise up toward the ceiling.

- Extend the crown of your head forward and reach back strongly through your heels to fully extend your spine.

- Look at the floor about six inches in front of your hands to keep the back of your neck nice and long.

- Engage your abs by drawing your navel up toward your spine.

- Stay here and breathe for five to ten long, slow, deep breaths.

Modifications:

◎ If holding this pose more than a breath or two is too challenging, lower your knees to the floor.

Benefits:

◎ Strengthens the entire body—arms, legs, back, stomach— giving you the stamina you need to break through old habits and make changes

◎ Builds heat in the body, fostering your inner fire (And fire is transformational—it burns off impurities and turns up the flame on your will to change.)

Other Remedies to Try:
Center of Power Stimulation
Cobra Pose • Ring the Gong

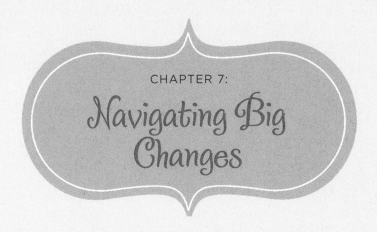

CHAPTER 7:

Navigating Big Changes

Thus far, this book has concentrated on remedies for specific situations of limited duration—a kind of triage for daily life. But inevitably, we'll all experience times of intense change that last for days, weeks, or even months, whether it's moving, having a baby, or losing a loved one. While you could fill an entire book on coping mechanisms for any one of these events, choosing even one simple practice to do during a major transition can be a powerful tool.

Spending a small amount of time each day performing the same self-care technique helps you stay simultaneously rooted and open, so that you can remain true to yourself as your life changes all around you and still flexible enough to grow into your new reality. It also gives you a way to take your temperature on a daily basis. Setting aside a few minutes each morning or night to practice a little self-care is the equivalent of asking your inner self how it's feeling and then handing it a microphone. If, in the third Sphinx Pose of your move, you notice that your shoulders are clearly achier, you'll know to take it easy for a day or two before tackling that next stack of boxes that needs to be unpacked. Or, if you're pregnant and keep falling asleep in Side-Lying Corpse

Pose, you'll (hopefully) realize that you need more sleep. It's all a means to open up a dialogue between your body and your mind so that you can use this time of transition to get to know yourself even better. May it be the beginning of a beautiful friendship.

Moving

Now that you're sitting there surrounded by boxes, not entirely sure where your underwear is, you remember why moving is widely considered one of life's most stressful events. Packing up everything you own and creating a new home for yourself—it's enough to shake anyone down to their roots.

The flip side of all this uncertainty is that you're inviting all manner of new things into your life—neighbors, routes to work, favorite coffee shop, and restaurants. You want to balance the need to ground yourself with an openness to change so that you can enjoy the infusion of new energy instead of feel overwhelmed by it. This pose is grounding, because you're literally down on the ground, but it also helps you look to the future and teaches you how to give yourself the support you need to navigate big changes. Practice it for a few minutes each night before bed during the transition, and maybe, just maybe, this will be your most painless move yet. ❁

Remedy:
Sphinx Pose

Ingredients:
Five feet of clear floor space with something cushy—
such as carpet, a yoga mat, or a towel—to lie on
Bare feet

Time Needed:
Five minutes

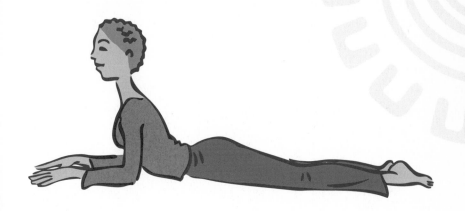

Instructions:

◎ Lie on the floor on your stomach.

◎ Bring your feet a little wider than hips' distance apart and tuck your toes under.

◎ Prop your torso up on your forearms with your elbows directly under your shoulders.

◎ Look straight ahead.

◎ Stay here and breathe for up to five minutes, allowing your heart to melt farther and farther forward as you release your buttocks and encourage your lower back to lengthen down toward your feet.

◎ Lower your torso down to the floor and rest, lying on your stomach with your head turned to one side, for a few moments before getting up.

Modifications:

◎ You *can* do this pose while watching TV. Of course, it's preferable for you to be in a quiet room or listening to soothing music to provide further relaxation. But if you're either going to do it while watching TV or not do it all, by all means, watch away. Just no channel surfing!

Benefits:

◎ Stretches the abdomen and stimulates digestion, counteracting the effects stress may be taking on your stomach

◎ Restores the natural curve in your spine at the lower back, making you better able to support yourself and stay supple during a hectic time

◎ Squeezes the adrenal glands, the stress hormone-producing glands located just above your kidneys in your mid-back, bathing them in fresh blood, regulating their function, and making you better able to handle stress

◎ Strengthens and stretches the muscles of the back, counteracting all the heavy lifting you've been doing

◎ Opens the chest and heart, helping you stay open to change

Other Remedies to Try:
Cobra Pose • Rescue Remedy
Supported Child's Pose

Getting Married

There's no doubt that being engaged is a magical experience. You've found the person you want to spend the rest of your life with and, miraculously, that person also wants to spend the rest of his with you. You've publicly declared your love and devotion to one another, which is exhilarating. And you've immediately become the center of attention, flitting from party to menu tasting to ring shopping where everyone fawns over you. With all of the activity and attention, you want to look and feel your best so that you can take it all in (and so you'll look great in all those pictures that will now be peppering your bookshelves and the walls of your parents' house).

Underneath all the merriment lies an undercurrent of immense stress. Everything is outlandishly expensive. You and your fiancé have differing tastes or priorities. And suddenly everyone in your family is acting really weird and making demands that don't jibe with your vision of your day. You have to stand up for yourself and grow up in a major and very public way, and growth is rarely a comfortable process. It's bewildering and sometimes painful—even more so when you're doing too many things, eating and drinking too much, and not sleeping or resting well.

> *Underneath all the merriment lies an undercurrent of immense stress.*

This remedy can give you a regular way to stop the madness and do something that eases your nerves as it restores your energy level. Do it every day, any time you feel the need to take a step back from the planning whirlwind. ✿

Remedy:
Legs Up the Wall

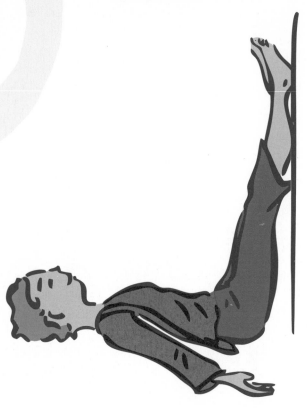

Ingredients:
Three feet of clear floor space next to a wall
A folded blanket or firm cushion (optional)

Time Needed:
Up to ten minutes

Instructions:

◎ Sit on the floor with your legs straight out in front of you and your right hip and shoulder grazing the wall.

◎ Bend your knees and bring the soles of your feet to the floor a few inches in front of your booty.

◎ Roll onto your left side, keeping your feet and your seat close to the wall.

◎ Now roll onto your back and straighten your legs so that they rest on the wall.

◎ Either place your palms on your stomach, extend your arms out to your sides (palms up), or bend your elbows ninety degrees and rest your arms on the floor with your elbows approximately even with your ears.

◎ Breathe and relax here as long as you feel comfortable, up to ten minutes.

◎ To come out, bend your knees and slide your feet down the wall. Then roll to one side and rest in the fetal position for a moment before pushing yourself back up to sitting.

Modifications:
N/A

Benefits:

◎ This pose manages to be energizing *and* relaxing. Because your legs are higher than your heart, your circulatory system doesn't have to work so hard to get blood from your feet back to your heart. Giving yourself a break from this constant need is extremely restful to the body as a whole, and the heart in particular.

◎ This reversal of gravity (which is what causes wrinkles, after all) and the increase in circulation gives you a glow that no makeup product can replicate.

◎ This remedy reduces leg strain and any swelling in the legs and ankles—all the better to help you dance the night away and look fabulous while doing it.

◎ It also stretches the hamstrings and the muscles of the lower back, alleviating many minor backaches.

◎ Finally, it quiets the nervous system and the mind so you can focus on taking in this major life event instead of merely getting through it.

Other Remedies to Try:
Cobra Pose • Rescue Remedy
Supported Child's Pose

Having a Baby

You can buy cute maternity clothes, continue working, and pretend to the outside world that everything is status quo. But despite your best efforts to appear "normal," pregnancy is an arduous undertaking. While you're experiencing it, you not only deserve special care, you require it.

Your body is not your own anymore, at least for the time being. There are many things you can't eat or drink, your digestion is out of whack, your energy level isn't what it was, you're peeing every ten minutes, and your silhouette is changing by the day. Mentally, you're on a hormonal roller coaster that has you glowing about the thought of meeting your new baby, in a tizzy about redecorating or de-cluttering, and irritated when your partner breathes on you—often all within seconds of each other. Just as your body has increased needs for calories, nutrients, and hydration, you also have an increased need for rest, pampering, and support. This remedy allows you to give yourself all three of these vital components of a healthy pregnancy in one restorative exercise.

You not only deserve special care, you require it.

Important note: Be sure to lie on your left side. There's a major vein, known as the inferior vena cava, that runs along the right side of the spine and carries blood from the lower half of your body back to your heart. When you lie on your right side, the baby can rest on the vein and impede blood flow from the lower half of your body and to the baby. Lying on your left side keeps the baby clear of the inferior vena cava and promotes blood flow throughout the body. ❧

Remedy:
Side-Lying Corpse Pose

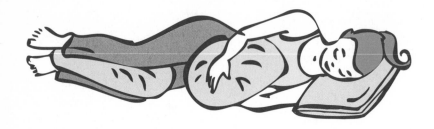

Ingredients:
Floor space
Comfortable clothes
Thin blanket
Two firm pillows, small couch cushions,
or yoga bolsters

Time Needed:
As long as you have, up to fifteen minutes

Instructions:

◎ Fold your blanket up into a compact pillow for your head.

◎ Have your cushions nearby as you lie on the floor on your left side.

◎ Place the blanket under your head to support your head and neck.

◎ Bend your knees and rest them on the floor at the same level as your hips. Place one cushion between your legs to support your right knee, shin, and foot.

⊚ Bring the other cushion to the floor in front of your chest and drape your right arm on it.

⊚ Extend your left arm under the cushion that's supporting your right arm.

⊚ Rest here, breathing normally through your nose and allowing your body to simply melt into the floor or your cushioning.

⊚ Focus your attention on the sound of your breath and let go of the need to do anything else—whether that's planning the nursery or scratching your itchy belly.

Modifications:
N/A

Benefits:

⊚ Babies you through this major—and exhausting—rite of passage

⊚ Deeply restorative, which is more important than ever now that your body is charged with creating and sustaining another life in addition to your own

⊚ Teaches you one way to make yourself comfortable at a time when few positions feel truly good

⊚ Quiets your mind, alleviating any mental drama you may be experiencing

Other Remedies to Try:
Ground Flaxseeds • Hot Ginger Tea
Listen to Your Body
Supported Reclining Bound Angle Pose

Getting Divorced

You fervently believed you'd be spending the rest of your life with this person but, alas, it's not to be. As with any ending, it's time to grieve your loss so you can usher in a new phase of your life with an open heart. It's easy to say, but harder to do. Grieving is scary. And at this very moment you're feeling wounded, possibly rejected, and a little adrift—not the mental state you want to be in when you're embarking on the rest of your life. What if you're inherently unlovable? What if starting over turns out to be more than you can handle? What if you can't trust your judgment and will never fall in love again? There are so many unknowns. Maybe it's easier just to hide under the covers.

Give yourself the sense of security and loving care you need with a daily self-massage. It may sound indulgent, but this practice has been heralded for thousands of years by practitioners of Ayurveda—the ancient school of medicine from India. Known as *abhyanga* in Sanskrit, the daily massage is seen as an important way to care for the body and the spirit. Everyone needs loving touch in their lives, and since you're in a wonky place where you are likely not feeling your most loveable, you can benefit from the deeply comforting effects of massage even more than the average person. Of course, it's lovely and worthwhile to pay for a professional massage, but if you can't give yourself the love and care you need on a regular basis, how can you expect someone else to do it for you? Treating yourself to the benefit of a massage administered by the most important person in your life—that would be you—is a great way to start healing your broken heart and get ready to head out into

> Give yourself the sense of security and loving care you need with a daily self-massage.

the next chapter of your life. It's free, it makes you feel tended to, and it gives you a metaphorical and physical glow—just what you need to light your way. Plus, it feels *really good.* 🌸

Remedy:
Self-Massage

Ingredients:
Massage oil (preferably organic)
An old towel

Time Needed:
Five to fifteen minutes

Instructions:

🌀 Gently warm your oil by holding it under a stream of hot water for several seconds.

🌀 Take off your clothes and jewelry and take a seat on your towel.

🌀 Pour a small amount of oil in your palm and start your massage at your head. Dump the oil on the top of your head and use your finger pads to work it throughout your scalp.

🌀 Massage some of the excess oil onto the outsides of your ears, your face (don't rub too hard here, as the skin on your face is delicate), all sides of your neck, your shoulders, and upper back.

🌀 Dot some more oil along your arms and rub it in using long, sweeping strokes over your upper and lower arms and circular motions over your elbows and wrists. Give each hand and your fingers some attention, too.

🌀 Use circular motions to rub more oil into your chest and abdomen. Use a clockwise motion over your stomach, as that's the direction your large intestine works and rubbing it in this way will encourage your digestion.

🌀 Treat your legs the same way you did your arms—long strokes on the thighs and calves, and circles over the hips, knees, and ankles.

🌀 Finish up by spending some time rubbing oil into your feet.

🌀 If you have time, sit quietly for a minute or two to let the oil penetrate.

🌀 Use your towel to wipe off any excess oil before showering or hopping in the bath.

Modifications:

🌀 You can use a wide array of oils: almond, sesame, coconut, or olive oil; or one of these oils mixed in with a few drops of your favorite essential oil; or a pre-blended oil that's marketed as "massage oil."

🌀 You can either give yourself a brief massage every day before your morning shower, or a longer massage once a week. While a daily massage is preferable—because you need love, attention, and touch on a daily basis, after all— if once a week is all you can manage, do it and don't feel guilty. It's much better than no massage at all.

Benefits:

🌀 Relaxes and gently stimulates so you can shed excess stress and help keep yourself from falling into a pit of lethargy

⊚ Provides a way to give yourself the love and attention you deserve and are likely craving at this time

⊚ Feeds your body from the outside in, providing moisture, nourishment, and warmth

⊚ Promotes detoxification, helping you slough off whatever you don't need anymore like a snake shedding its skin—the perfect accompaniment to the rebirth you're experiencing

⊚ Can help keep your skin supple and less likely to wrinkle and sag as you age, if you can develop a regular habit out of it

Other Remedies to Try:
Awkward Pose • Rescue Remedy
Supported Child's Pose
Supported Heart Opener
Warrior's Breath

Losing a Loved One

O n some level, everyone knows that death is an inevitable part of life. But when someone you love dies, this knowledge does very little to shelter you from the emotional roller coaster of grief. At this most vulnerable time of your life, when you're nursing a wounded heart and reckoning with your own mortality, you need an infusion of tender loving care. And while friends, family, therapists, and spiritual teachers can all provide invaluable support, you also have an important role to play in your own healing.

Tend to your broken heart with a practice based on the premise that what you focus on grows stronger. Just like dwelling on a problem will make it loom larger, spending a few moments a day concentrating on your physical and metaphysical heart will nourish it and help it mend. It also ensures that you don't bury your feelings, which, although tempting, leads to numbness and feelings of isolation—two states of being that will only extend this undeniably difficult time and make it even more challenging. By focusing on your heart, you'll send the part of your self that's hurting the most the message that there is hope. ✤

Remedy:
Heart Meditation

Ingredients:
Privacy
Comfortable seat

Time Needed:
As little as a few seconds to as long as fifteen minutes

Instructions:

- Sit somewhere you feel safe and comfortable.

- Rest both palms on your heart.

- Close your eyes.

- Breathing normally, focus on your chest. Feel the weight of your hands resting there, the breath flowing in and out, and perhaps even your own heartbeat.

- If it comes easily to you, visualize your heart starting to glow (just like E.T.!)—vibrant, radiant, and whole.

- Spend as long as fifteen minutes reveling in the concept of your own heart keeping you alive, connecting you to others, and holding a spot for your loved one.

Modifications:

- Although formal heart-centered meditation is beneficial, so is checking in with your heart throughout the day. As you brush your teeth, walk to work, drive to lunch, and cook dinner, take a deep breath and imagine vitality and warmth surrounding your heart.

- If you check in with your heart and feel numbness, pain, or another unpleasant sensation, don't fret. Simply notice what you feel and don't make any attempts to wish it away. When you can be honest with yourself about how you're feeling, your emotions will be much more likely to shift on their own accord. You'll also know much more about what you need to do to feel better.

Benefits:

◎ Heart meditation builds energy in your heart chakra, which yogis believe is the source of love, compassion, self-acceptance, and the ability to connect with others— all things that will help ease your journey through grief.

◎ Even if it feels like nothing is happening, something is. By taking the time and attention to focus on your heart, you are building your ability to love and be loved. The changes may be subtle, but over time, they will help you find your way out of grief.

◎ This exercise builds your ability to feel sympathy for and understanding of yourself and others, which will help you be gentle with yourself as you heal and truly connect with others who can help you during this difficult time.

> **Other Remedies to Try:**
> Supported Child's Pose
> Supported Heart Opener
> Warrior's Breath

Dealing with Injury or Illness

The news from your doctor isn't good. Whether it's an injury or an illness, your health is being challenged and it's time to gather all your resources—mental, physical, and otherwise—and prioritize getting better. Clearly, the advice of medical professionals will be invaluable now. But you also have an important role to play in your recuperation. Finding even one simple thing to do each day that tends to your physical and emotional needs will help you stay steady in the weeks, months, and years to come. Consider incorporating this restorative twisting exercise into your daily routine as a simple way to nourish your inner self as well as your physical self. After all, you'll need a resilient spirit as well as a healthy body in order to meet this challenge.

Twists keep your spine flexible and relaxed and can help you make any changes your illness will require of you with grace. They also encourage the body to eliminate waste and toxins so you can better shed whatever isn't working for you. This particular twist, with its outstretched arms and broad chest, also encourages more vitality-enhancing oxygen to flow into your lungs and wards off the depression that so often accompanies a sunken chest. And because this twist is supine, it also helps you build more time for more rest into your busy life and proves to your inner self that you are making well-being a priority.

> You need a resilient spirit in order to meet this challenge.

As many people who have lived through them will tell you, health problems often have lessons to teach about making more room for what's most important to you and letting go of things that don't serve you. By creating time for a regular self-care practice, no matter how simple, you signal your body that you are open to hearing what it has to tell you. And when your body knows you are listening, it won't have to speak quite so loudly with aches, pains, and other symptoms to get your attention. May this pose speed your journey to a full recovery. ✿

Remedy:
Knee-Down Twist

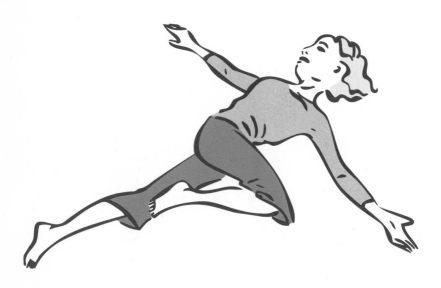

Ingredients:
Clear floor space
Pillow (optional)

Time Needed:
Five minutes (two minutes or so on each side)

Instructions:

🌀 Lie on your back on the floor with your legs straight and your arms extended out to your sides at shoulder height.

🌀 Draw your right knee into your chest and lightly rest your right foot on your left knee.

🌀 Allow the right knee to fall across your body and come to rest on the floor outside your left thigh.

🌀 Your right shoulder will want to follow your right leg and pop up off the floor; keep guiding it back down. It may not stay on the floor, but coaxing it down will help your chest stay as broad as possible.

🌀 If it's comfortable, turn your head to look at your right fingertips.

🌀 Stay here and breathe deeply for two minutes.

🌀 As you breathe, imagine creating as much space in your torso and spine as possible. Let your hips twist more deeply to the left as your shoulders grow more and more rooted into the floor.

🌀 After two minutes, return to the starting position, then repeat with the left leg.

Modifications:

🌀 You can make this pose extra comfy by doing it in bed, either in the morning before you get up, at night before you fall asleep, or both. To really make it decadent and cozy, place a pillow under your bent knee (if that feels good to you).

🌀 Turning your head to look at your opposite hand extends the twist all the way up to the very top of your spine. But if it causes any twinges in your neck, simply look up at the ceiling.

Benefits:

🌀 Wrings stress out of the spine and the muscles of the back and helps your entire back be more supple and resilient

🌀 Compresses the abdominal organs, encourages the elimination of toxins, stimulates digestion, and promotes the flow of fresh, oxygen-rich blood to the area

🌀 Opens the chest and encourages breathing to deepen, which is relaxing and revitalizing

🌀 Provides a simple way to tend to your body's changing needs as well as a guaranteed time-out for your mind as you go through a stressful time

---

Other Remedies to Try:
Sphinx Pose • Supported Child's Pose
Supported Heart Opener
Warrior's Breath

Epilogue:
If You Want to Go Further

Say you've tried a few of the remedies in this book and you've noticed that they actually do help you feel better—even if it's just the tiniest bit. You're intrigued by all this self-care stuff and are beginning to wonder how much better you could feel on a regular basis if you did more of it. Here are some simple ways to move a little further down the path. It doesn't really matter which route you decide to follow, only that you heed whatever part of you is telling you to take the next step. Happy trails.

Start a Practice

To take your self-care efforts out of the realm of triage and make them a regular component of your life—one that helps you stay on a more even physical and emotional keel and makes you less likely to need triage in the first place—consider establishing some sort of mind-body practice. I define a practice as, "What you do with regularity even when you don't feel like doing anything at all." It could be something formal, such as tai chi, yoga, or meditation, by all means. But it could also be something much more freeform and uncomplicated, such as walking, needlepoint, painting, baking bread, or some other hobby. It can also be a combination of things—say, one yoga class a week and gardening, or knitting each night before bed and two mornings of tai chi. Whatever activity you choose, it should be something that makes you feel the best version of yourself—grounded, clear, generous, and calm. A regular practice gives you an outlet to process your daily life, creates an opportunity for your clearest thinking to rise to the top, and gives you a reliable touch point to help you stay steady during rocky times.

There are only two major requirements of a practice. First, it should involve your mind and your body, even if it's not necessarily exercise. There is something about requiring your mind to focus on some action in your body that takes you off the endless treadmill of worry and stress and creates an opening for calm and balance to take their place. The other requirement is that it be something that calls to you. Don't let your practice be something you feel you "should" do. This is your opportunity to indulge the part of yourself that longs for something more than the daily slog. If you have an unexplained interest in Chinese calligraphy, pursue it. When you heed the call of your inner voice, it will lead you where you need to go.

If you choose a formal discipline, start looking around for classes and/or teachers. If you're interested in yoga, for example, take yourself on a yoga safari: commit to checking out a new class each week or so until you find one with a teacher, ambience, and time that feels right to you.

And perhaps most important, remember: Although you do want to give yourself over completely to whatever activity you choose whenever you do it, there's no need to be perfect. It is called "practice," after all. You only need to keep showing up.

Set a Balance Benchmark

Another helpful tactic is to establish a balance benchmark for yourself—a sign that helps you make sure you're headed in the right direction. Because balance is fluid, a constant process of assessing and recalibrating, the work of staying on track never ends. (I apologize for delivering this disheartening news.) But you can leave a trail of bread crumbs for yourself to help ensure that you remain on the path to wellness.

A balance benchmark is a simple yet fulfilling activity that makes you feel calmer and happier, even when the rest of your life is a chaos factory—kind of like a practice, but with less formality. My balance benchmark, for example, is eating one home-cooked meal a day. Because I work from home and love to cook, the goal is fairly easy—a crucial component of a valuable benchmark. But some days, the list of things to do and the number of interruptions pile up to the point where taking ten minutes to scramble some eggs feels like too much. When it's a once-in-a-while occurrence, I fix a bowl of cereal and get back to the stove the next day. But when two or three days have passed without my dirtying a pot, I know I need to cut back on my obligations.

Your balance benchmark can be any activity that you enjoy deeply. It could be attending a weekly stitch n' bitch, reading before bed, devoting ten minutes a day solely to playing with your pet, or drinking a cup of tea each morning in your favorite chair—your choices are endless. But do pick just one benchmark. The idea is to build a little breathing space into your daily schedule, not crowd it with ever more things you simply must do.

Learn to Speak Your Body's Language

This last piece of the self-care puzzle is much more about listening than doing. We all have our recurring symptoms—whether it's an ulcer that keeps coming back, a case of eczema that continually flares, a back muscle that's prone to spasm, or a propensity toward migraines. It's a common human response to notice that you're getting another cold sore, or back ache, or headache, and feel defeated and frustrated—how could this be happening again? But there is another way to respond to these chronic ailments. Think of them as your body's way of communicating.

When your perpetual symptom flares up, take it as a sign that your body is saying, "I need you to pay attention to me, or else." And you really don't want to find out what "or else" means. Better to notice that a cold sore is blooming and cancel your plans for the night, make some soup, and go to bed early than continue at your frantic pace and wind up with a massive scab that lasts for three weeks. It won't necessarily make your cold sore immediately disappear, but it will quell some of the conditions that triggered it in the first place and boost your body's ability to fight it. It may seem decadent. But you at your best is always more valuable than you just slogging through.

I'm not suggesting that your troublesome ailments aren't worthy of medical attention, or that they are figments of your imagination. I personally have a stiff neck that seizes up on me every once in a while when I am getting overwhelmed by daily life, and I can promise you, it hurts. But the sooner I recognize that it is coming on, the more quickly I can respond with some quiet time, a massage, and more time spent on the yoga mat. Although the pain still comes periodically, the time between outbreaks is longer and the stiffness now fades much more quickly. And that's the beauty of taking time to listen to your body and having an array of self-care tools at the ready—the better you get at recognizing your body's signals, the more subtle your adjustments can become.

The Dalai Lama teaches that we should consider anyone who causes us pain to be a spiritual teacher. You can apply this logic to your body as well, and begin to see your nagging ailments as a little angel on your shoulder, nudging you to take better care of yourself. The more you learn to respect your body's whispers, the less work you'll have to do to respond to them. Perhaps you'll even get to the point where you'll be able to recognize nonphysical challenges—whether it's a rocky patch in your relationship or a boss who leads by terrorizing—as an opportunity to make changes for the better rather than something to be simply endured. By listening to your body, treating yourself to a regular self-care practice, and making sure you don't veer too far off the road to balance, you'll be much more open to whatever life brings.

Appendix:
Reading List and Other Resources

Absolute Beauty: Radiant Skin and Inner Harmony through the Ancient Secrets of Ayurveda (Harper Perennial, 1997), by Pratima Raichur with Marian Cohn

Explains how to look (and feel) your best using Ayurveda, covering everything from diet and exercise to product recommendations for your particular constitution. Best of all, she runs a spa, called Pratima, in Soho in New York City. It's definitely worth a visit if you are in the area!

Acupressure for Emotional Healing: A Self-Care Guide for Trauma, Stress & Common Emotional Imbalances (Bantam Books, 2004) ***and Acupressure's Potent Points: A Guide to Self-Care for Common Ailments*** (Bantam, 2000), both by Michael Reed Gach., Ph.D. (***Acupressure for Emotional Healing*** co-authored with Beth Ann Henning, Dipl., A.B.T.)

These books are very comprehensive and easy-to-understand guides to using acupressure to relieve common ailments. Gach is the founder of the Acupressure Institute in Berkeley, California. He also runs acupressure.com.

Bringing Yoga to Life: The Everyday Practice of Enlightened Living (HarperOne, 2005), by Donna Farhi

One of my favorite books, this title explores the myriad ways a regular practice of yoga can change your life for the better, and inspires you to keep committing to your self-care practice, whatever that may be.

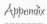

Consciously Female: How to Listen to Your Body and Your Soul for a Lifetime of Healthier Living (Bantam, 2004), by Tracey W. Gaudet, M.D., with Paula Spencer

Dr. Gaudet is one of those rare doctors who combines the best of Western medicine with the wisdom of Eastern practices. This book discusses what it truly means to be a woman and will also teach you a wide array of powerful tools you can use to open a dialogue with your body and vastly improve your health and overall sense of well-being.

Faith: Trusting Your Own Deepest Experience (Riverhead, 2003), by Sharon Salzberg

Salzberg is a meditation teacher, but this book isn't about learning a particular style of meditation. Instead, it teaches how to cultivate your awareness of your own state of mind to enrich your life. Non-dogmatic, easy to comprehend, and deeply touching, Salzberg's stories will inspire you to wade a little further into the mindfulness waters.

Herbal Healing for Women: Simple Home Remedies for Women of All Ages (Fireside, 2003), by Rosemary Gladstar

You know chamomile tea can soothe an upset stomach, or that lighting a lavender-scented candle helps you relax. Now learn about some of the hundreds of other herbs you can use to keep your mind and body on an even keel. Gladstar also provides great perspective on how diet, lifestyle habits, and emotions affect our health, making this book an invaluable tool for any woman who's interested in taking full responsibility for her health and well-being.

***The Miracle of Mindfulness: An Introduction to the Practice of
Meditation*** (Beacon Press, 1999), by Thich Nhat Hanh
Hanh, a Buddhist monk from Vietnam, is the equivalent of a living Gandhi. During the Vietnam War, he traveled to America to speak against the war and promote nonviolence—an effort that forced him into permanent exile. Undaunted, he has continued to work with veterans of all wars, promoting peace through meditation. His teachings are brief, but they are profound. This is a great book to dip into whenever you need to remind yourself how powerful peacefulness can be.

Natural Choices for Women's Health: How the Secrets of Natural and Chinese Medicine Can Create a Lifetime of Wellness
(Three Rivers Press, 2005), by Laurie Steelsmith, N.D.
A comprehensive guide to navigating all of the major phases of a woman's life from a naturopathic doctor who also incorporates treatments from traditional Chinese medicine.

***The Woman's Book of Yoga & Health: A Lifelong Guide to
Wellness*** (Shambhala, 2002), by Linda Sparrowe and Patricia Walden
I practically sleep with this book under my pillow. It contains clearly illustrated yoga sequences geared to help you with a wide variety of physical conditions, including headaches, backaches, eating disorders, pregnancy, and menopause. An invaluable resource.

www.MsMindbody.com
My own Web site, where I send out a weekly newsletter that covers one simple technique you can do to master the fine art of feeling better and better. MsMindbody members are also constantly sharing their self-care tips and supporting each other on our quest to feel a little less frazzled and a little more fulfilled. I'd be honored to have you join us.

Index

About the Author

KATE HANLEY is a writer and certified yoga teacher who specializes in exploring the mind-body connection. She is a contributing editor at *Body + Soul* and writes regularly for *Natural Solutions*, *Delicious Living*, LHJ.com, GoodHousekeeping.com, and iVillage.com. She lives with her husband and daughter in Brooklyn, New York, and can be found online at www.MsMindbody.com.

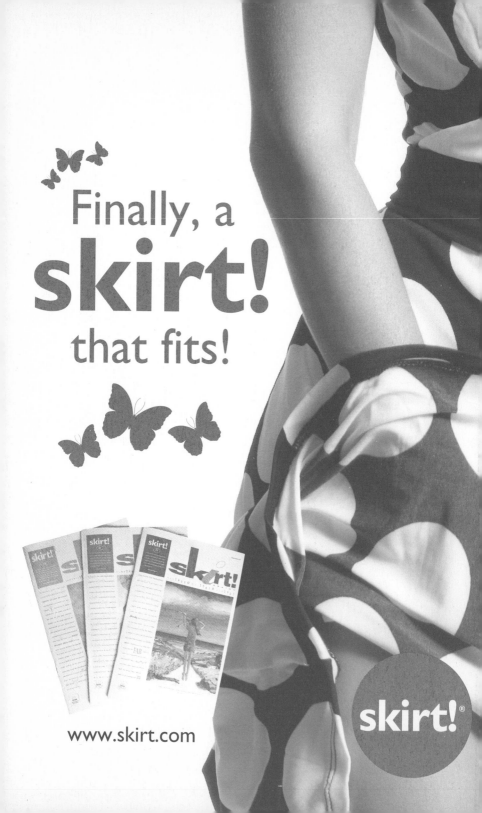